STRAIGHT TALK
WITH YOUR
GYNECOLOGIST

*How to Get Answers
That Will Save Your Life*

Eddie C. Sollie, M.D., OB/GYN
Author

Peggy Clarke
executive director, American Social Health Association
Foreword

Sara Steinberg
Contributing Editor

Beyond Words Publishing, Inc.

Published by
Beyond Words Publishing, Inc.
13950 NW Pumpkin Ridge Road
Hillsboro, Oregon 97123
Phone: 503-647-5109
Toll-free: 1-800-284-9673

Developmental Editor: Julie Livingston
Page Layout: The TypeSmith
Cover Design: Soga Design

Printed in the United States of America

The information contained in this book is intended to be educational
and not for diagnosis, prescription, or treatment of disease or of any
health disorder whatsoever. This information should not replace
competent professional advice and does not guarantee that a person
will not contract a sexually transmitted disease. The contents of this
book are intended to be used as an adjunct to a competent sex- or
STD-education class. The authors and publisher are in no way liable
for any use or misuse of the material.

ISBN 0-941831-83-3

Dedication

To those people past and present who inspired me to write this book: my loving wife, Cindy; my beautiful daughters, Erica and Andrea; my parents, Dr. and Mrs. David Sollie; my mentor, Pelham Staples, M.D.; and Diane, whose needless death should remind all women of their rights and responsibilities to participate in their own health care.

Acknowledgments

Years ago when my patient, Diane, suggested to me that I write a book, I knew I could not do it alone. What I did not know was that all kinds of wonderful and supportive people from many different walks of life would lend themselves to this project. I wish I had space enough to acknowledge them all.

My special appreciation, then, to Sandy Nelson, long-time friend and co-worker; Jan Miller, my agent; Sara Steinberg; Peggy Clarke, executive director of the American Social Health Association; Dan Scott, M.D., and Presbyterian Hospital of Dallas; and all the nurses and patients who generously shared their emotions and experiences with me. Thanks also to Julie Livingston for her editorial contribution. Last but not least, my gratitude to my publishers, Richard Cohn and Cindy Black, and their staff at Beyond Words Publishing.

Contents

Foreword

Talking about your sexuality can be one of the most difficult things to do. Despite the plethora of television talk shows, situation comedies, and soap operas that focus on the issue of sex and highlight the drama and trauma of personal relationships, Americans are reluctant—and unprepared—to examine and discuss their own sexual behavior. Yet it is precisely frank discussion of sex that increases the likelihood of satisfying relationships and makes for healthier sex lives. In fact, it is arguable that communication about sexual health is essential to our overall health.

Many people are unaware of the important link between how we behave in the bedroom and our general physical well-being. Even in the era of AIDS, with stories about this tragic epidemic appearing in the media every day, a surprising number of people have not thought about its implications for themselves. Even more surprising are the millions of Americans who have never heard of the array of other sexually transmitted diseases that threaten our lives and those of our loved ones.

Each year in this country, twelve million people are infected with a sexually transmitted disease. The great majority acquire these infections unknowingly, often from partners who do not know that they are harboring the infections. Despite the fact that these diseases are spreading rapidly throughout our society, many people continue to believe that sexually transmitted diseases are "other people's" problems—until it happens to them.

Every day, thousands of men and women call the American Social Health Association's national hotlines with questions about infections they thought could only happen to other people. Many of them had been under the mistaken impression that their heterosexuality somehow protected them from exposure to an infection. For others, the fact that they are currently in a monogamous relationship gave them a false sense of security about disease. The reality of a diagnosis brings home the sad truth that any sexually active person can acquire a potentially harmful infection.

Women are disproportionately affected by sexually transmitted diseases, and yet they, too, are reluctant to discuss this important topic. A couple's discussion about sexuality needs to be frank and direct. We need to put aside our embarrassment or concern that by starting the conversation, we might give the other person the wrong impression. Open discussion about sexuality and personal safety can only help relationships. And when the risks of infection are faced and dealt with, sexual experience can be more fulfilling, as well as much healthier.

Caring communication between partners is a major component of sexual health. Communication between a patient and her health care provider is also an essential aspect of achieving and maintaining good health. Yet here, too, many women are reluctant to raise important questions about their sexuality with their doctors. Perhaps the connection between our private sexual activity and our physical health is not clear to everyone, but the fact that what we do affects how we feel, demands that we talk openly with the people who care for our health.

The relationship between a woman and her gynecologist must be based on a shared goal: achieving and maintaining the patient's optimal health. Toward that end, both the physician *and* the patient must openly communicate about all matters affecting the patient's well-being.

Let's face some truths here. If talking about sex with our partners is difficult, discussing sexual behavior with our doctors can seem an impossible task. Visits to the doctor's office can be nerve-racking. The office environment is generally unfamiliar, the procedures aren't always clear to us, and the examinations are uncomfortable. And, since doctors are supposed to look for signs of problems we don't want to have, even routine checkups can generate anxiety. Reluctance to discuss intimate behavior under these circumstances is understandable, but this reluctance must be overcome.

Women need to seize the opportunity offered during medical checkups to take an active role in protecting their health. By viewing the relationship as a partnership—or a shared responsibility to optimize the patient's well-being—women can move out of a passive, submissive role into a productive, active stance in which their knowledge and their actions can positively impact their future.

In this book, Dr. Eddie Sollie provides a blueprint for women to build positive partnerships with their doctors. This book holds the answers to many long-held questions and concerns about personal health. It also makes the important link between sexual behavior and overall health—a long-overlooked connection essential to optimal health care. Dr. Sollie unveils the rationale behind every aspect of a typical visit to the gynecologist's office. He explains the approaches physicians take to providing basic health care and challenges women to become active participants in these services. From a doctor's perspective, Dr. Sollie reveals the complexities of discussing sexual health and emphasizes their relevance by recounting poignant professional experiences. Most importantly, he emphasizes, again and again, the importance of open communication between women and their doctors.

Dr. Sollie's book demonstrates his sensitivity to patient's concerns and his philosophy that physicians must share information and decision making with their patients. His book is a tool that will facilitate women in assuming their rightful role in this relationship. Armed with the realization that sexual health is an important component of overall health, women can follow the straightforward advice of this caring physician as they establish better communication with their own doctors.

—Peggy Clarke, executive director,
American Social Health Association

Why Should You Read This Book?

Here's a simple quiz to help you decide:

1. Have you ever had sex—even *once*—in your life?
2. Do you ever intend to have sex?

Did you answer yes to either of the above questions? If you did—regardless of your lifestyle or your age, no matter whether you are married or single, currently celibate or in a monogamous relationship—this book could save your health, your fertility, the health of your future children, even your life. Despite all the attention that has been focused on HIV and AIDS, a multitude of other, "silent" epidemics that primarily afflict women are going virtually unnoticed. I am talking about sexually transmitted diseases (STDs).

*"But I'm not the kind of woman who gets **those** diseases!"* Is that how you respond, deep-down, when you hear about STDs? That is a dangerous attitude. STDs are a much more serious health threat than most women realize, and they happen to one out of every four women between the ages of fifteen and fifty-five. Any woman who has sex, even *once* in her life, may unknowingly contract an STD that can threaten her sexual health and her life. Believe me, if you don't think a sexually transmitted disease could ever happen to you because you are a "nice" girl or woman, you are

in the highest risk group of all—you are a person who doesn't have the information you need to protect yourself.

"Why haven't I heard about these epidemics?" Unfortunately, you may already have contracted and been treated for an STD *without ever being told that you had one.* Many women diagnosed with an STD are kept in the dark about what they have. They are treated for "infections" or "pelvic pain" that "somehow just got there," never knowing that their condition stemmed from an STD. Also, some widespread and health-threatening STDs have few or no symptoms that patients can detect, yet most gynecologists do not routinely screen for them. Women just like you have suffered needlessly from STDs. You will meet some of these women in the pages of this book—they have courageously shared their ordeals with complete candor. They deserve to be heard, and you owe it to yourself to learn from their experiences.

You may have a hard time believing some of what you're going to read. Parts of it will probably anger you, but that is not my intent. This isn't meant to be a negative book or a doom-and-gloom warning—not at all. This book will sound an alarm, but keep in mind that gynecologists seldom encounter immediate, life or death emergencies. We will be talking about serious problems, but they are problems you can learn about and take steps to prevent.

Why shouldn't you simply leave all this in the hands of your doctor? No matter how much you like your gynecologist, and no matter how well qualified he or she* is, your first line of defense against this health threat is not your doctor—it is YOURSELF. You need to become an informed

---

* I recognize that gynecologists, like everyone else, come in two models: male and female. However, since many of the issues I will address are specific to the relationship between a female patient and a male physician, I will use the masculine pronoun most of the time. Where appropriate, I will use the feminine pronoun.

consumer of health care, so that in the doctor-patient relationship, you will be aware of your rights and your responsibilities. I want to educate you and empower you to take responsibility for protecting your own health. When you need a gynecologist's help with prevention or treatment of disease, I want you to be the kind of patient who stands up for your right to receive the best care available.

As you read this book, imagine that I am your gynecologist and that you and I have set up a confidential appointment in which I will answer any and all questions. You can have as much of my time as you need. Best of all, you aren't going to have to take your clothes off, and there won't be a physical examination; so you can relax.

The purpose of this meeting is to work together as equals—members of the same team—to protect your health. And that means the two of us will talk *straight* with one another. You'll give me all the information I need to give you the best possible care, and I will answer *every one* of your questions in terms you can understand. We'll settle back in comfortable chairs behind closed doors and communicate frankly and honestly.

Much of what we're going to talk about, few people discuss openly. If we could really sit face to face and talk, you might feel embarrassed at times. You may find this hard to believe, but many doctors feel the same way. We know more about medical science than you do, but we were raised in the same society as you were, and we don't shed all our hang-ups just because we have M.D. degrees. So you don't have to feel embarrassed about *being* embarrassed.

If we were talking one-on-one, you might also feel embarrassed about asking what you think are silly or stupid questions. There is no such thing as a stupid question when your health depends on getting complete information from your doctor. *Not* asking all your questions doesn't sound very smart, does it?

In reality, unless you are a patient in my own practice, I can't sit across from you. I can't coax you into opening up and asking your questions, and I can't hold your hand to help you get through any emotions that surface. But if you'll stick with me through these pages, I'm going to talk to you as if you *were* my patient, and we are going to work together to arm you with the knowledge you need to protect your health.

Since I don't know how much you know about your own body, I'm going to cover things on an elementary level. Most women today are much better informed about health issues than their grandmothers were, but everyone has gaps in basic knowledge. Learning that one crucial fact you didn't know before could safeguard your health, even your life. I'm not going to talk down to you, but I am not going to assume that any important information is already common knowledge. I won't try to impress you with my command of scholarly writing. Along the way I'll explain the medical terminology you must know to ask your doctor the questions that are crucial to your health, but I intend this book to be an "easy read," not a textbook.

By the way, there's no rule that says we can't smile or laugh together. A healthy sense of humor is a constructive way to approach any problem.

In the Introduction, you will meet a perfectly respectable, intelligent woman who could have been easily and inexpensively treated for the STD she contracted, if only her doctor had been honest with her. The medical nightmare she went through as a result is shocking because it happens so often to so many women and because it stems from a simple lack of information.

Part One will begin to give you that information. First, you need to know just what I mean when I say that engaging in sex—even once—involves serious risks to your health. For sex to be truly pleasurable, it has to be as worry-free as possible. But before you can reduce the risks involved, you have to know what they are. In other words, if you're going to be sexually active, you need to do it with your eyes open, knowing all the possible consequences. Chapter 1 (which details these risks) may hold some surprises for you: you may not have known that some of the most widespread health problems for which women seek treatment are caused by sexually transmitted diseases.

In Chapter 2, I'll explain what I mean when I say that women are being kept in the dark about the "silent" epidemics of sexually transmitted diseases that are raging through all levels of society. We'll explore how this lack of information becomes a roadblock to the prevention and treatment of STDs.

Part Two will prescribe a cure for this information gap: an equal partnership, based on respect, between gynecologists and their patients. My goal is to enable you to create this kind of doctor-patient relationship in your own life. This section includes specific advice on how to find the right gynecologist for you, how to obtain second opinions, and how to gain access to your medical records. An entire chapter focuses on how you can get the most out of the gynecological examination. I have put special emphasis on the Pap test: how it should be conducted, how and why you must learn to read the actual lab test results for yourself, and what you need to know if any abnormalities show up.

In short, Parts One and Two contain the most important information in this book, because they will empower you to ask the questions that can save your health and your life. The remainder of the book will instruct you in detail as to specific questions to ask.

Part Three starts with a general introduction to sexually transmitted diseases. Since the typical gynecological exam does not routinely screen for most of these, individual chapters will cover the information you need on the STDs that are most widespread today. Armed with this knowledge and with the questions you need to ask, you will be in a better position to help your doctor help you.

What do you need to know and what actions should you take if you contract an STD? Part Four prepares you with the questions you'll need to ask your physician; it also includes advice on getting a second opinion and exercising your right to have access to your medical records.

Since a large percentage of gynecological surgeries are related to diagnosing or treating STDs, Part Four concludes with a chapter on how to prepare for outpatient or hospital-based surgical procedures. This section will coach you on the questions to ask ahead of time and how a surgical patient deserves to be treated.

Prevention of sexually transmitted diseases gets special attention in Part Five. Along with basic information, this section focuses on how you can choose, discuss, and practice prevention strategies with your partner.

Please don't overlook the information in the Appendix, which is meant to be as "user-friendly" as possible. Here you will find a glossary of terms, and a listing of resources for more information, along with a section for young women.

I asked you to think about why you should read this book. With all I have just said, I still can't help you answer that any better than to tell you the story of a woman I know who contracted a sexually transmitted disease. Many of my patients have shared their own stories through this book, giving freely of their time so you could hear about STDs from a woman's point of view. In the Introduction that follows, I would like to tell you about one of these courageous women. It is because of what women like her have gone through that you hold this book in your hands.

Introduction

Diane* had everything going for her. A bright, eloquent, and beautiful woman of twenty-two, she enjoyed her job as an executive secretary and was looking forward to her wedding. By middle-class American standards, she was a respectable young woman with a promising future.

Experiencing a vaginal discharge, Diane sought care at a nationally known women's clinic. When the results of her Pap smear came back negative, Diane was given a cream to relieve her symptoms. But when her discharge did not clear up, she started asking questions. Could her problem have anything to do with a small growth on her fiancé's penis? The clinic gave Diane a second Pap smear and some antibiotics and assured her that her fiancé's little bump had no direct or indirect relationship to her symptoms.

Six months and several visits after she had first reported her symptoms to the clinic, Diane began experiencing abnormal vaginal bleeding. She had also developed exterior genital warts. Her symptoms were now too serious to be treated at the clinic, and they referred her to me. I was able to see her right away, but it was too late. A biopsy showed she had a highly aggressive, invasive form of cervical cancer.

Diane could not have known that her original Pap smear had been incorrectly read as negative by one of the worst labs in the country. But she should have been told that the

---

* To protect their privacy, I have changed the names of all patients whose case histories appear in this book.

clinic's own findings indicated there were lesions on her cervix. She should have been told that her second Pap smear revealed precancerous cells.

Apparently no one wanted to offend such a "nice girl" by telling her that her lesions were due to genital warts—a sexually transmitted disease. They didn't offend her, but their "good manners" cost her her life because certain forms of genital warts are the leading cause of cervical cancer.

Diane went through radiation, multiple surgeries, severe weight loss, and many months of hospitalization before she died. The worst part was that none of it made any sense. Why hadn't the clinic told her that her second Pap test indicated a problem? Why was she given antibiotics when the clinic's records showed they knew she had a condition caused by a virus (human papilloma virus, or HPV) that never responds to antibiotics? When she asked about her fiancé's symptoms, why hadn't she been told he needed treatment? In short, after seeking care and asking questions, why hadn't she been told the truth about her condition?

Perhaps the clinic staff didn't want to think lovely, respectable Diane could have that "stupid little wart" that supposedly only "bad" girls get. Over the years, I have treated a number of call girls, and most of them are too streetwise to get a sexually transmitted disease. In fact, they are pretty good diagnosticians of STDs because their livelihood depends on good sexual health. They come in every few months to be tested for every disease in the book; they understand the risks and take precautions to avoid them. It is women like Diane who usually pay the price for ignorance about STDs. How sad to be killed by a myth: "nice" girls don't get "those" diseases.

Diane's fiancé is paying the price, too. He lost the woman he was going to marry, and the guilt that he feels is almost unbearable. He blames himself because a virus he carried caused the death of the woman he loved.

How could Diane's death have been prevented? If the clinic had tested her for genital warts during her gynecological exam, she might have lived. If she'd had enough education about sexually transmitted diseases to suggest that her fiancé get checked out, she might have lived. If she'd known enough about the threat of STDs to practice "safer sex" methods, she might have lived. If she'd insisted on getting the results of her second Pap smear—asking to see the actual laboratory report—she might have lived.

Diane's was not a rare case, and the issue goes way beyond the fact that gynecologists and other health professionals sometimes show poor judgment in withholding important information from patients. My contention is that every woman has the *right* and the *responsibility* to educate herself about any potential threat to her health, including STDs, and to stay informed about her own medical condition. This is what I mean by being a partner with your physician. How to achieve that partnership is the focus of this book.

Through the long months of her battle against cancer, I grew very close to Diane. I felt much anger over the needlessness of her death, until she taught me anger wasn't effective. Before she died, she begged me to take action so that other women wouldn't have to die from sexually transmitted diseases. "Eddie, you have a big mouth," she said. "Tell other women. Put it in writing so I won't have to die again and again and again."

And so this book is for Diane, and for all the other women you will meet in these pages, "model patients," who rarely questioned anything their doctors said and who thought that an STD would never happen to them. Most of all, it is for you.

Educate yourself and open your eyes. Although STDs may have seemed invisible to you before, chances are they have already touched your life or the lives of people you know. They are linked to "abnormal" and precancerous Pap smear results, to cervical cancer, to pain during intercourse, and to pelvic inflammatory disease (PID); they are linked to many cases of infertility; they are linked to ectopic pregnancies. They are often the reason that you or women you know have been given antibiotics for "pelvic infections" or have undergone biopsies, laparotomies, laparoscopies, colposcopies, cryosurgeries, laser surgeries, and hysterectomies.

I want to give you the knowledge, the tools, to take charge of your own life. If you're going to be sexually active, then not knowing how to talk straight with your doctor or not knowing the facts about STDs makes about as much sense as crossing an expressway at rush hour with your eyes closed. If you are willing to open your eyes, you'll find you don't have to cross that street alone. I want you to have a healthy and pleasurable sex life! Your allies can be this book, a gynecologist of your own who is a partner in your wellness and—most of all—an educated, informed consumer of health care: YOU.

Let's begin our new partnership by taking a look at a few facts you probably never knew about sex and your health.

PART ONE

CHAPTER 1

"I Never Knew Sex Could Cause *That*!"

Some health risks linked to sex that might surprise you

When I asked you to consider why you should read this book, I promised to talk straight with you. I'm going to start right now. If you want to stay healthy and continue to enjoy your life as a woman, we need to begin with an honest, un-flinching look at the health risks involved in being sexually active. You have to be willing to learn about them and to admit when they apply to you. If it turns out that none of these risks apply to you, terrific! The knowledge you'll gain might help someone you know—even your own daughter.

Before I get more specific, I would like to address those of you who are married. Are you safe from AIDS and other sexually transmitted diseases (STDs) because you are mar-ried? There are no 100 percent guarantees, but you are almost certainly safe if you've been married to the same per-son since the late 1970s (when the AIDS virus first appeared in the United States) and your marriage has been absolutely monogamous and neither of you has used intravenous (IV) drugs or received blood transfusions during that time.

You are *not* entirely safe if you and your spouse have been married for a few years and you've been absolutely faithful to one another and don't use IV drugs. Why? Because you both have a past. I'm sure you've heard that it may take from eight to eleven years after a person is infected with HIV—the virus that causes AIDs (see Chapter 6 for more information)—for AIDS symptoms to show up. Men and women can also harbor any of the other sexually transmitted infections in their bodies for years without any symptoms, unknowingly passing them on to their sexual partners.

The good news is, if you both get tested for the sexually transmitted diseases I will describe, test negative or get treated for any STDs that are found, and remain mutually monogamous as well as drug-free, your marriage can be a life raft that takes the two of you safely through treacherous waters. Education is essential if you are to achieve good health. You must also be tested properly for all the STDs that pose a threat to your health.

Unless you've been living on a deserted island for the last decade, you've heard about some of these risks. How do you feel about the information you've gotten? Before you answer, take a look at an imaginary patient I'll call Jane. Do you share any of her views?

Jane thinks back with nostalgia to the "good old days" when a woman's only concern during her childbearing years was the chance of unwanted pregnancy. She knows that STDs have been around for a long time, though in her parents' and grandparents' days they were called venereal diseases (VD). Jane always thought of VD as the scourge of prostitutes, drug addicts, and extremely promiscuous people. She also recalls the stereotypical image of soldiers watching VD training films on the perils of associating with "loose" women.

Jane tries to keep up with what's going on in the world, so when AIDS and HIV came on the scene, she followed each new development. She formed her strongest impressions about AIDS in the early days when it seemed to threaten mainly homosexuals and IV drug users. Back then Jane had compassion for the plight of these people, but she didn't feel personally threatened by the epidemic. If AIDS was being spread through promiscuous sex and the sharing of drug needles, she reasoned, this was self-destructive behavior that people could choose to change. The true victims in her eyes were children who contracted AIDS in the womb and people who received contaminated blood transfusions. Jane now understands that many people contracted and became carriers of HIV long before they knew the threat even existed. She knows the virus is spreading into the heterosexual community, but she still views AIDS as a disease of promiscuity.

In recent years, Jane has begun to hear about other sexually transmitted diseases. She is concerned about their impact on society and follows media reports on them with some interest. In fact, she finds it challenging keeping up with the flow of information. Almost every day brings a new study or report that seems to contradict what she heard the day before. Some of the diseases, such as chlamydia and genital warts, were new to her at first. She also learned that many of the diseases she still associates with the VD label— syphilis, gonorrhea, and herpes—are on the rise.

Intellectually, Jane knows that most of these so-called other STDs are much more widespread than AIDS. They are so widespread, in fact, that if they were strains of the flu, Jane would probably feel concerned enough to ask her doctor about the availability of a vaccine. Yet, because these diseases are sexually transmitted and Jane isn't the kind of woman who "sleeps around," in her mind they happen only to other people.

Jane is dangerously misinformed. There are so many ways she can unknowingly contract an STD and go about her life unaware that it's doing damage inside her. There are also many ailments that Jane's gynecologist might treat her for without telling her that she contracted them sexually. In Chapter 2, we'll look at why STDs are such a "hidden" epidemic, and why not knowing that you have an STD is extremely hazardous.

Before we talk about the added danger of not knowing you have a sexually transmitted disease, I will cover the basic risks of contracting one. If you choose to engage in sexual activity these days (and remember, this even applies to a one-time-only sexual encounter) and if, as a result, you come down with a sexually transmitted disease, what could happen to you?

That is a complicated question because there are more than twenty-five different kinds of STDs, and some of them overlap in the medical problems they cause. We'll wait until Part Three to take a really comprehensive look at each of the most common STDs. For now, I will give you an overview of the health risks STDs pose. We'll divide our discussion between causes and effects—a cause, for example, being an individual STD like hepatitis B, and an effect being a syndrome like pelvic inflammatory disease (PID, which is caused by several different STDs, sometimes singly, sometimes in combination). We'll put aside for now those STDs that are more annoying than dangerous. However, we'll want to run through all the STDs that pose a threat to pregnant women and newborns.

You've probably heard about most of the diseases and medical problems we're going to cover, but you may not have associated some of them with sex. You'll notice that the risks these problems pose fall into four basic groups. They are 1) the risk of death, 2) the risk of becoming infertile, 3) the risk of death or serious medical complications to your newborn child, and 4) the risk of chronic illness. We could also talk about the inconvenience, discomfort, and expense of undergoing surgical and other procedures to diagnose and treat STDs, but we'll give those topics the in-depth treatment they deserve in Chapters 4 and 17.

HIV and AIDS

Risks and/or consequences:

- Eventual death from the failure of the immune system to protect the body from infection
- Eventual death of many children born to infected mothers

Any discussion of the health risks associated with being sexually active has to start with AIDS. You may feel you've been bombarded with reports on the epidemic of HIV and AIDS, but please stay with me here. I'll save the detailed information for Chapter 6, but here are the most important things you need to know about the risks to you:

Infection rates are soaring among women. In 1992, nearly half of all new AIDS victims worldwide were women. In the United States, the epidemic is spreading the fastest among women, especially those who have used drugs intravenously or whose partners are currently using or have done so in the past. AIDS is among the top five causes of death of U.S. women of childbearing age. By the year 2000, the World Health Organization projects that almost 50 percent of new AIDS infections will be among women.

AIDS is becoming a heterosexual epidemic. Heterosexual women are increasingly becoming infected through intercourse with infected men.

Many women with AIDS aren't diagnosed early enough to take advantage of treatments that could prolong their lives. Sixty-five percent of women who die of AIDS are not properly diagnosed prior to their deaths.

AIDS is a time bomb. Just because you have remained free of AIDS until now, you should not feel at ease. In every gynecologist's practice there are women just like you who are not and have never been promiscuous, and who have never knowingly slept with an AIDS-infected person or with anyone in a high-risk category (hemophiliacs, homosexual or bisexual men, and IV drug users). But remember, when you sleep with someone, you are also sleeping with all of their past partners, and all of their past partners' partners, and so on. If you feel safe because you have been with the same partner for several years, remember that many HIV-infected people have gone for as long as ten years without having recognizable symptoms. An HIV-infected person is contagious during this incubation period even though he or she looks and feels fine.

Pelvic inflammatory disease (PID)

Risks and/or consequences:

- Death from rupture of a tubal (or ectopic) pregnancy or rupture of an abscess
- Infertility due to scarring of the reproductive organs
- Hysterectomy, with removal of the ovaries—early menopause—in serious cases
- Chronic suffering from pelvic pain
- Serious medical complications in newborns

If you have ever been treated for "pelvic pain" or "a pelvic infection," you were probably being treated for PID. This is an infection of the female reproductive organs. The infection starts in the cervix, moves into the uterus, then spreads to the fallopian tubes and ovaries. It leaves scar tissue, or adhesions, that can block the fallopian tubes and damage other reproductive organs.

PID is most often caused by sexually transmitted diseases that have gone untreated, especially gonorrhea and chlamydia (see Part Three). Other STDs that can cause PID include nongonococcal urethritis (NGU), mycoplasma, and ureaplasma. If a doctor tells you that you have an infection that was caused by "a little virus" or "just a little bacteria," insist on knowing the exact name of the disease. Most of the diseases that cause PID have names, and there are ways of diagnosing them. Knowing what is involved in your case makes a difference in the medical treatment you and your partner should receive.

Probably the best-known medical emergency caused by PID is a pregnancy in the wrong place—a tubal, or ectopic, pregnancy. If scar tissue blocking a fallopian tube prevents a fertilized egg from reaching the uterus, the egg implants itself in the tube. When the growing egg ruptures the tube, a woman can bleed to death unless she has emergency surgery.

Frequently, a PID infection can cause an abscess, or an accumulation of pus, in the abdomen. These abscesses can be difficult to treat with antibiotics. It's rare, but I have seen women die from ruptured abscesses.

PID is very often the culprit behind infertility; scarring of the fallopian tubes blocks the egg from getting through the tube to be fertilized. Most of us know someone who had to undergo surgery to open blocked fallopian tubes, or even extensive surgical reconstruction of the pelvis. PID caused by a sexually transmitted disease is frequently the reason couples seek costly in vitro fertilization procedures.

Infertility is more than just a medical risk; it is emotionally devastating to learn that you can never bear children. Having children may be the furthest thing from your mind right now, but the time may come when you want a child, and you may be unable to do so. Let us hope that never happens to you. If it does, I hope you won't have to go through the added regret of realizing there were warning signals you ignored that could have gotten you to the doctor in time to save your fertility.

PID doesn't always lead to infertility. Many women who have had PID achieve wonderful, healthy pregnancies, but the scarring in their pelvises may cause chronic pelvic pain. These women are also constantly sore and usually uncomfortable during intercourse. If their male partners try to tell them that pain during intercourse is not that bad, I suggest they ask their partners to imagine how they would feel if someone were to squeeze their testicles really hard every four or five minutes. That's the kind of pain a woman can experience when PID goes undetected.

If PID is left untreated for a long time, the resulting scarring or adhesions can become so extensive and painful that hysterectomy—and sometimes the removal of the ovaries (oophorectomy)—is the only option. Imagine the catastrophe of this happening to you at a young age: Not only will you never bear children, but you will experience hot flashes (because your ovaries have been removed) unless you take hormones for the rest of your life.

What are the symptoms of PID?

Depending on the kind of sexually transmitted disease that caused your PID, it can take anywhere from several days to several months for PID to develop. In the early stages, up to 80 percent of women with PID show no symptoms at all. Even if you have early symptoms, they can be so mild that you might ignore them. PID often starts with abdominal pain that feels like a bad menstrual cramp but isn't helped by the pills you usually take for cramps. You might have a discharge that doesn't look or smell normal. Pain during intercourse and painful urination are also warning signals. Although you probably won't have a fever right away, you might feel nauseated. You may still be able to go to work or school, but you just won't feel right. That's the time to see your doctor for testing to prevent the complications I've described.

Be attuned to your body. If you suspect that something is wrong, trust yourself. Don't ignore these symptoms, because while you're thinking they're all in your head, they can be eating up your fertility.I recall one young woman who came to see me complaining of frequent cramps. Her previous doctor kept telling her she merely had a bad case of gas or constipation. When I eventually performed surgery on her, I found that both of her fallopian tubes were scarred. Her "constipation" was PID.

If you ignore the early symptoms of PID, you won't be able to ignore them later on. By the time you have serious PID, you'll hardly be able to walk. You'll have what we call the "PID shuffle." You'll walk in short little steps because it hurts so much to move; when you sit, you'll feel your insides are hurting and burning. You'll probably also have a high fever. If you wait until you feel this way, you probably will have damaged your fertility and need hospitalization.

To recap, a woman with PID might have none, some, or all of the following symptoms:

- Pain in the lower abdomen resembling severe menstrual cramps
- Unusually painful or heavy periods
- Vaginal bleeding between menstrual periods
- Pain during intercourse
- Pain during urination
- Nausea and/or vomiting
- Fever
- Lower backache
- Abnormal vaginal discharge

Who is most likely to get PID?

Since most cases of PID are related to sexually transmitted diseases, the more sex partners you have, the higher your risk. Women in their teens who have multiple sex partners are at greatest risk because their reproductive organs are not completely mature, making them less resistant to infection. If you are using an intrauterine device (IUD) for birth control and are exposed to an STD, the microorganisms could travel up the IUD string into your uterus. Also, if you have had PID before, you are more likely to get it again if you are reexposed to STDs such as gonorrhea or chlamydia.

Do men show symptoms of the infections that cause PID?

Men can't get PID because it's a disease of the female reproductive organs; but men can get the STDs that cause PID and can pass them on to their partners. Although men are more likely than women to have STD symptoms, in about half of all cases men are symptomless. The most visible symptoms in males are a pus-like discharge from the penis or pain and burning during urination. Men with these symptoms should seek treatment right away to keep from passing on to their partners an infection that could cause PID.

Can PID be cured?

Antibiotics will cure the infection. In severe cases your doctor may need to hospitalize you and administer antibiotics intravenously. Sometimes the damage PID has already done to the reproductive system can't be repaired, but if you go to your doctor at the first signs of PID, chances are good that you won't end up infertile or in the hospital, and you won't need a hysterectomy.

For more information related to PID, see Chapter 7 on chlamydia and Chapter 9 on gonorrhea.

Dysplasia and cervical cancer

Risks and/or consequences:

- Eventual death from precancerous cell changes (dysplasia) if left untreated
- Hysterectomy or partial hysterectomy
- Reduced fertility or infertility resulting from diagnostic or treatment procedures
- Early menopause if ovaries are removed or damaged during treatment

Has someone you know ever had a series of abnormal Pap smears or been treated for precancerous cells of the cervix (dysplasia)? Did the doctor perform "a little laser surgery?" Did she do a cone biopsy or use cryosurgery or heat cauterization to destroy the abnormal cells?

You probably know that preventing cervical cancer is the goal of all these procedures. Cervical cancer is the second most common cause of death from cancer among women worldwide. But did you know that cervical cancer is an infectious disease that is almost always spread through sexual intercourse? Did you know that the culprit behind cervical cancer is usually HPV, the human papilloma virus, a widespread sexually transmitted disease? The vast majority of abnormal Pap smears that require treatment are caused by this virus, and it's closely associated with 90 percent of all invasive cervical cancers.

There's also a strong link between genital warts and the development of cervical neoplasias, abnormal growths that often become cancerous. Genital warts are caused by a subtype of HPV but not necessarily the one that causes cervical cancer. More than 40 percent of the U.S. population now has the virus, although many don't have visible symptoms. In Chapter 2 I'll tell you why some patients aren't told they are being treated for genital warts, and I'll cover genital warts in greater detail in Chapter 8.

If I have visible genital warts, am I likely to get cervical cancer?

Although there are more than seventy different types of HPV, the kinds we're talking about do not cause warts on the hands and feet; they are transmitted only through vaginal, oral, or anal sex. Certain strains of HPV have been linked with precancerous growths, which can become cancerous without treatment. These lesions can appear on the cervix, in the vagina, on the labia or vulva, or on the anus.

Genital warts aren't always visible, even when they grow on the outside of the body. HPV can produce microscopic warts that are visible only with the help of special instruments, or can live in the skin without causing warts at all. As I said earlier, the strains of HPV that usually cause visible genital warts are not the strains that are most closely linked to cancer. However, since HPV causes genital warts and has been found in the cervical cells of nearly all women with cervical cancer, you should consider genital warts a risk factor for cervical cancer.

Who is most likely to get cervical cancer?

We estimate that about 60,000 women in the U.S. develop cervical cancer each year, and some 7,000 to 10,000 women die of invasive cervical cancer each year. Cervical cancer is the second leading cause of death due to cancer in women.

Cervical cancer acts like a sexually transmitted disease: your risk of cervical cancer is directly related to the number of sexual partners you have had, and how young you were when you began having sex. You are at higher risk for the disease:

- If you have had multiple sexual partners
- If your partner has had multiple sexual partners
- If you became sexually active before age eighteen (because immature cervical cells are more vulnerable)
- If you have a history of vaginal infections, genital warts, or genital herpes
- If your mother took DES (diethylstilbestrol), a synthetic hormone widely prescribed between 1940 and 1971 to prevent miscarriage
- If you had your first child before age twenty or have had many pregnancies
- If you are a smoker or are regularly exposed to secondhand smoke

Although the number of deaths from cervical cancer has dropped by 70 percent since the Pap smear was first introduced in 1943, we are currently worried about an observed upswing of cases in women under thirty-five. At least one-quarter of all invasive cervical cancer now occurs among women as young as seventeen. Since the early 1960s, cervical cancer in teens and young women has increased by more than 150 percent. It also appears that younger women are susceptible to an especially aggressive form of cervical cancer that can develop as soon as a year or two after they have had a negative Pap smear.

The good news is, we know now how to prevent the majority of cervical cancers, and we know how to treat the virus before the cancerous process begins. That's why it is so important for you to know about HPV and other cervical cancer risk factors and to have regular pap tests.

In Chapter 4 I'll talk about how to interpret your Pap smear report. The Pap smear does not directly detect HPV infection. However, if you have an abnormal Pap smear, the report will tell you how far along the abnormality has progressed, and whether the lab found the kind of cell changes usually associated with genital warts. Chapter 8 will cover genital warts as an STD in great detail—the cause, as opposed to the effect. For now, let's focus on the effect, the usually slow progression from precancerous changes to cervical cancer.

When normal, healthy cells in the cervix undergo abnormal changes in their size, shape, and number, we call these lesions dysplasias. This isn't cancer, but it can develop into very early cancer. Dysplastic cells resemble cancer cells under the microscope, but they don't invade nearby healthy tissue. Dysplasia is classified as mild, moderate, or severe, and it develops most often in women between twenty-five and thirty-five years of age. These cells should usually be removed, although in some mild cases they return to normal without treatment.

The earliest form of cervical cancer we can detect—what we call carcinoma in situ (meaning in its original position)—involves only the top layer of cervical cells. It can stay in this layer for many months, even years. This very early cervical cancer develops most often in women between thirty and forty years of age. When detected and treated at this stage, cervical cancer is nearly 100 percent curable.

Cancer that invades deeper layers of cervical tissue is called invasive cervical cancer. It usually takes from eight to thirty years for dysplasia to develop into invasive carcinoma. When caught at this stage, the cure rate is still about 85 percent. But if the cancer spreads to nearby tissues or organs, that figure drops to 30 percent. With a further spread to the lymph system and blood vessels, the five-year survival rate is only 10 percent. Invasive cervical cancer usually occurs in women between the ages of forty and sixty.

What are the symptoms of cervical cancer?

Unfortunately, dysplasia and early cervical cancer rarely cause any symptoms. In the later stages of cervical cancer, symptoms can include:

- Vaginal bleeding between periods
- Vaginal bleeding after sexual intercourse or douching
- Menstrual bleeding that lasts longer and is heavier than usual
- Foul-smelling, often bloody discharge

Can cervical cancer be cured?

Yes, if caught early. If all women had pelvic exams and Pap smears regularly, most cervical abnormalities would be detected early enough to be treated effectively.

For more information on the various diagnostic and treatment procedures your doctor is likely to recommend if your

pelvic exam and Pap test detect any problems, see Chapter 4.
For more information on genital warts, see Chapter 8.

Syphilis

Risks and/or consequences:

- Death
- Stroke
- Tumors
- Blindness
- Heart disease
- Insanity
- Nervous disorders

A lot of people think of syphilis as a disease of drug addicts, prostitutes, and the urban environment in general. While syphilis is still rare compared to other STDs, it is on the upswing. Reported cases have doubled since 1984, with 150,000 new infections reported yearly. As recently as 1988, syphilis rates reached their highest level in forty years. Syphilis is one of the few STDs that is life-threatening to both men and women.

It takes many years for syphilis to become lethal, and although antibiotics can stop the disease at any stage, they can't reverse damage already done. Unfortunately, syphilis is difficult to detect in its first and second stages, after which it remains dormant for ten to twenty years until it reaches the deadly third stage, when the time bomb goes off.

I know this sounds scary, and it is. But if syphilis is caught early, an inexpensive injection of penicillin or other antibiotic can stop it. Fortunately, a simple blood test can detect this disease.

For more information on syphilis, see Chapter 11.

Hepatitis B

Risks and/or consequences:

- Cirrhosis of the liver
- Liver cancer
- Permanent liver damage
- Long-term fatigue
- Death

"Hepatitis" means inflammation of the liver, and hepatitis B is the virus strain that causes this kind of hepatitis (which is also known as serum hepatitis or long-incubation hepatitis). Hepatitis B isn't usually thought of as a sexually transmitted disease, but sex is its leading mode of transmission. Unfortunately, many people never know they have hepatitis B and become chronic carriers, passing it on unknowingly to their sexual partners. This is one reason why cases rose 67 percent between 1978 and 1985, even though a vaccine was introduced in 1982. Since the 1980s, hepatitis B has been on the upswing among heterosexuals.

When the virus attacks the liver, the patient usually suffers severe fatigue, nausea, vomiting, loss of appetite, headaches, and general body aches. Jaundice, a yellowing of the skin and the whites of the eyes, sets in a few weeks later. The fatigue and flu-like symptoms can make a patient miserable and interfere with her daily activities for up to four months.

While there is no cure for hepatitis B, most people recover naturally. Unfortunately, if your liver is damaged, you will experience the side effects of the disease (especially chronic fatigue) for the rest of your life. About 5 to 10 percent of patients have severe liver damage, and some 5,000 Americans die of hepatitis B every year.

Since hepatitis B is the only viral STD that we can treat with a vaccine, it's ironic that so few people are aware of the disease. Fewer than one percent of all heterosexuals who are at risk for hepatitis B have taken advantage of the vaccine.

For more information on hepatitis B, see Chapter 12.

Risks STDs pose to pregnant women and newborns

HIV and AIDS

As the rate of infection increases in women, we'll see a corresponding rise in the number of children born who are infected with HIV. More than one-third of all babies born to HIV-infected women become infected during pregnancy or at delivery. Most infected infants die before age three.

Pelvic inflammatory disease (PID)

Some of the sexually transmitted diseases that cause PID can also endanger newborn children. See especially chlamydia and gonorrhea (following).

Chlamydia

Chlamydia, which causes an estimated 50 percent of all PID cases in this country, can afflict a newborn with pneumonia, ear and respiratory infections, an eye inflammation called conjunctivitis, and low birth weight. The mother also runs increased risks of having a stillbirth, a premature birth, or postpartum fever.

Genital warts

If warts are present at the time of delivery, there is a slight chance that you could pass them on to your child, causing complications such as an infection or the growth of warts in the baby's throat. You might even need a cesarean delivery, because sometimes the hormones of pregnancy stimulate the warts to bleed or to grow large enough to block the birth canal.

Gonorrhea

We've already talked about gonorrhea as one of the two main causes of PID, but it can also cause a crippling form of arthritis called Reiter's syndrome in adults (characterized by joint pain, eye inflammation, and skin sores). Gonorrhea can infect a child's eyes at birth, causing blindness. For this reason, the eyes of newborns are commonly treated with either silver nitrate or an antibiotic to protect them. Many infants also develop infections of the vagina and rectum, as well as pneumonia or other complications.

Pregnant women with gonorrhea are also much more likely than uninfected women to have their amniotic membranes rupture prematurely ("breaking of the water"), causing premature delivery.

Genital herpes

Herpes simplex type 2 is more of an annoyance than a health threat in adults (as Chapter 10 will explain), but genital herpes poses great danger to a newborn. If the mother is experiencing an active outbreak during delivery, the child has a 50 percent chance of contracting the disease during its passage through the birth canal, and is at high risk of brain damage, blindness, or death. The doctor may recommend a cesarean delivery to prevent the virus from being passed on in this way. Neonatal herpes can also cause premature birth, fever, lethargy, skin and mouth sores, pneumonia, and complications of the nervous and other organ systems. Fortunately, a woman whose herpes is inactive will not pass it to her child during delivery. If a woman contracts genital herpes for the first time during the pregnancy (primary herpes), she faces an increased risk of miscarriage and premature delivery, because the first (or primary) episode of herpes is usually much more virulent than later outbreaks.

Syphilis

The greatest risk with syphilis is that an infected woman could unknowingly pass the disease on to her unborn baby any time after the fourth month of pregnancy. Congenital syphilis in children carries the risks of death, brain damage, blindness, bone or dental deformities, anemia and other blood disorders, extensive skin sores, and severe nasal discharge. Symptoms might appear at birth, or months—even years—later. Syphilis also poses a heightened risk of miscarriages, stillbirths, and prematurity.

Hepatitis B

An infected pregnant woman can pass this disease on to her baby with deadly consequences; 35 to 40 percent of these children die. Hepatitis B is so contagious that a woman who suspects she has been exposed should not breastfeed until she is checked out by a doctor.

Almost all of the diseases we've been discussing pose a greater risk to women. I know that isn't fair, but that's the way it is. Disease organisms have a much harder time getting through the many layers of skin cells on a man's penis. Not only can they pass more easily through the thin, delicate lining of a woman's vagina, cervix, and uterus—especially the immature cell lining in an adolescent woman—but that warm, moist inner environment is a much better breeding ground.

Men can carry around sexually transmitted diseases for years without ever having a clue as to their existence. Men rarely die from most of the illnesses caused by STDs. However, I know a man who unintentionally passed an STD on to his fiancée that ultimately caused her death (see Introduction). He is a man in pain and will be a victim of that STD for the rest of his life. Men don't run the risk of losing their chance to bear a child, but a man whose mate becomes infertile as the result of an STD is also a victim of infertility.

Men have fewer opportunities than women to become educated about the hazards of sexual activity because they don't have occasion to visit doctors as often as women see gynecologists. When a man wants something to use for birth control and protection against STDs, he doesn't see a doctor for a prescription—he can simply buy a condom. Women have been intensively educated about the value of a yearly gynecological exam; most men put off yearly examinations until they start getting concerned about their blood pressure and cholesterol levels.

My point here is that the information I have just presented on the health hazards of being sexually active is information that needs to get out to both men and women. Men and women share the pleasures of sexuality, so men and women should share the responsibility of understanding the hazards involved and taking steps to reduce them. If possible, invite your partner to accompany you to talk to your gynecologist about testing for STDs and preventive measures. If your partner won't go, then pick up written material that the two of you can read and discuss together. Above all, take responsibility for educating yourself and safeguarding your own health.

In the next chapter, we'll look at why—more often than you would think—many gynecologists don't tell women the vital fact that their medical problems are caused by a sexually transmitted disease.

CHAPTER 2

"Patient Does Not Know... Do Not Tell Her"

Withholding information is a gamble, and the stakes are your health or your life

Imagine that several weeks after your annual gynecological exam, you get a note in the mail on a Friday afternoon, informing you that you had a "bad" Pap smear. Alarmed, you try frantically to reach your doctor, only to hear that he won't be available to talk to you until Monday.

When that happened to Lesley, a married woman of forty, she lost confidence in her doctor and decided to find a new gynecologist. A friend referred her to Doctor X, who was a prominent physician of obstetrics and gynecology at a major metropolitan hospital. He assured her that he would never send a patient bad news via the mail. Lesley decided to see him every six months for a Pap test, to be sure that she would be carefully and closely watched.

Four years passed. Then, three weeks after her last checkup, Doctor X called to say that Lesley had a Class III Pap smear. (Class III refers to precancerous or severely abnormal cells. As we will see in Chapter 3, this classification method is being phased out in favor of a more descriptive system.) Doctor X performed a cervical biopsy on

Lesley, followed by laser treatment to destroy the pre-cancerous cells.

"I asked him why I turned up with precancerous cells when I had been visiting him so regularly," Lesley recalls. "There was no history of cancer in my family, and I was not sexually active before I married. His answer to me was 'It just happens.' He told me to keep coming for Pap smears every six months, but I said that wasn't good enough. I went every three months, because I thought I was coming to the end of my life. I was fearful, stressed out, and very depressed."

Doctor X also began recommending that Lesley have a hysterectomy. "He would never tell me why or what was wrong," says Lesley, "just that I was coming to the age where I might need a hysterectomy. For almost two years I was a nervous wreck, thinking that there were cancer cells in my body and wondering what to do."

Eventually Lesley told her story to a physician friend over dinner. He urged her to consult another gynecologist. I believe he had a strong hunch about what was going on, because when he called me about her, he said, "I think you'll be honest with my friend, no matter what the consequences are." So she came to see me, drumming her fingers and fidgeting, apologizing for feeling confused, and seeing herself as neurotic. She explained that she liked and trusted her doctor, and felt embarrassed to be switching practices.

In my examination of Lesley, I also found precancerous cells. She did need a hysterectomy. I asked her to get her records from Doctor X. "He says I don't need them," she reported back. She had to argue with him for several weeks before he released the records. We found out why when we looked through the stack of her lab reports.

In the very first report of an abnormal Pap, dated January 1986, there it was in black and white: condyloma. That's a fancy name for genital warts, our nation's most rapidly

spreading sexually transmitted disease (STD) and the leading cause of cervical cancer. Genital warts had caused
Lesley's precancerous cells, and the only way she could
have gotten the warts was through sexual relations with the
only partner she'd ever had, her husband. That prompted
Doctor X's lie "It just happens." Naturally, Lesley was ap-
palled, but the real shock came when we found hand-
printed instructions at the top of the lab report reading
"Doctor X said not to tell her."

On the report from her October 1986 Pap test, not only
was condyloma indicated once again, but the pathologist
had commented, "The cytologic abnormalities seen in the
previous smear persist." The report also recommended a
Pap smear be repeated in three to four months. And there
at the top of the chart, printed by hand, were the words "No
note sent—Patient does not know. Repeat in 6 months."

The further Lesley read, the angrier she became. Her next
Pap had been normal, but three months later, she tested
abnormal again. Three months after that, abnormal again.
Doctor X had never told her about those abnormal findings.
He had biopsied her at that point and given her laser treatment but had never informed her that he was treating her
for an STD.

Moreover, since Doctor X hadn't told Lesley that she had
genital warts, he failed to tell her that her husband also
needed to be checked. I explained to her that genital warts
don't always appear on the exterior genitals; males and
females can have the warts inside their genital organs, and
can unknowingly transmit them to a partner during intercourse. Unless both partners are treated, the warts usually
bounce back and forth between them like a ping-pong ball
(the same is true of many other STDs). A urologist con-
firmed that Lesley's husband did indeed have genital warts.

Why had Lesley's doctor withheld so much information
so critical to her health? Lesley presumes he was afraid that

the issue of sexually transmitted disease would jeopardize her marriage, and that husband and wife would accuse each other of bringing genital warts into the marriage through an affair (although her husband might just as easily have contracted genital warts before they met, then transmitted them to her after they were married). As it turned out, Lesley's husband did confess to an affair. However, Lesley and her husband are still married. They sought counseling, which is the responsibility of the patient. Our responsibility as doctors is to educate patients and give them the facts about their conditions.

Once Lesley learned the truth, she no longer felt neurotic; instead, she was furious. By keeping her in the dark, the doctor, whom she had trusted, had taken a gamble, letting her condition deteriorate until she was dangerously close to full-blown cervical cancer. She wrote a letter to Doctor X, which concluded by saying: "I would assume that a physician of your level would know that withholding medical information [from] a patient is unethical and bad medicine." Lesley is absolutely right, but unfortunately, withholding information from patients is not a rare practice.

Lesley did the right thing by asking questions, but she could not have foreseen that her doctor would lie to her. So what could she have done differently? First, she could have refused to accept vague statements about how abnormal cells "just happened" to appear. Instead, she could have asked to read the actual lab report for each of her Pap smears and requested copies of them. Then she could have asked her doctor to explain what the reports meant by *condyloma*.

That should have raised a number of other questions for Lesley to ask her doctor. But what if she didn't know enough about genital warts to ask all the important questions? What if, like many women, she would have felt embarrassed to ask questions pertaining to her sexual behavior? When a woman is facing a "bad" Pap smear or other upsetting news, she may not be in the right frame of mind to think of all the questions she should ask. This book will list those questions for you.

A patient who is an informed consumer asks a lot of questions, and that takes up more of a doctor's time. When doctors get together in the physicians' lounge of almost any hospital, some of them complain about this type of patient. But no doctor who has your best interests at heart will be offended if you bring a list of questions to your appointments to make sure you cover all the bases.

If Lesley asked but didn't get all her questions answered, she could have gotten a second opinion or even changed doctors. I know a lot of women find both these options very unpleasant, and many don't know the best way to go about finding another doctor. Chapter 3 will cover all these aspects of the doctor-patient relationship, empowering you to cultivate a partnership with your gynecologist based on open, honest communication.

Straight talk with your doctor can spare you the years of doubt and fear—capped by major surgery—that Lesley experienced. As she says today, "My doctor didn't tell me what was wrong because he obviously thought I was a neurotic and very nervous woman. But when I found out I had a sexually transmitted disease, it didn't ruin my life. Once I understood what happened and how it had happened, it set me free!"

What happened to Lesley, and even to Diane (whom you met in the Introduction)—being damaged by an STD their doctor never told them they had—could happen to you. In fact, it could already have happened to you! STDs, primarily those that cause cervical cancer and pelvic inflammatory disease (PID), are killing and seriously damaging women at what could be called epidemic levels. Many women don't even know they have these diseases, often because their gynecologists fail to inform them.

I assume you're going to need some convincing, because it's human nature to think that disaster always strikes someone else. Besides, why should you believe me, when this crisis isn't being widely announced in banner headlines or leading off the evening news?

A large number of my patients come to me with STDs or problems related to STDs; about 40 percent of the surgeries I do are the result of an STD. These numbers pertain only to gynecological care, as my practice does not include obstetrics. The situation in my practice is not unique; about one-half of all office visits to gynecological practices across the country are directly or indirectly related to STDs.

> I'm amazed at the number of physicians who have absolutely no idea how many new sexually transmitted infections occur each year. They haven't figured out how important it is. There's a denial there, just as there is a denial in some patients.
> —Peggy Clarke, executive director,
> American Social Health Association (ASHA)

It would be easy to say that these so-called other STDs are overshadowed by AIDS, but there's a lot more to it than that. Why isn't a public spotlight focusing on the epidemic of the other STDs when it clearly puts so many women at risk? Several reasons come to mind. The first and most obvious, discussed at the end of Chapter 1, bears repeating: almost all the other STDs endanger women, not men. Without dwelling on this issue, I'll ask you one question: How many women are in positions of power—in government, the mass media, the health care industry, and big business—positions that would enable them to aim that spotlight?

The other STDs have also been called a "silent" epidemic because the most serious of them have few symptoms a woman could detect on her own until the disease reaches an advanced stage. Genital warts, for example, can hide inside a woman's reproductive tract as well as inside a man's penis. Chlamydia usually causes no obvious symptoms until the complications of PID show up much later. You might assume that gynecologists routinely test for the most serious STDs during annual examinations, but you would be wrong. Many gynecologists don't even make patients aware that testing for STDs is available. It is your responsibility as a patient to request that your doctor test you for specific STDs. (You will pay extra for these tests.)

Undoubtedly, the hardest aspect to understand about this silent epidemic is how even the most well-meaning gynecologist—the one with the Marcus Welby-like bedside manner who may have been treating you for years—could fail to tell you that you had an STD. There is no single answer, but my experiences have shown me that the problem generally comes down to this: if your doctor sees you as a "nice" girl or woman, he may assume that you could not handle knowing you have what used to be called a venereal disease. He may think that he's protecting you from this information, but he's also protecting himself from having to break this kind of news to you.

That's an oversimplification of a complex situation, so I'd like to share with you the process I went through to reach this conclusion. Please bear in mind that I don't want to paint all gynecologists with the same brush. I am certainly not saying that every gynecologist fails to communicate important information to patients. All those who withhold information are different, and they do so for differing reasons. The more you know about those reasons, the better equipped you will be to take responsibility for becoming an informed patient.

When I think back to the days when I was a young doctor doing my residency training in obstetrics and gynecology, I remember that every time I arrived at the county hospital clinic to work my shift, I'd stare in disbelief at the overload of patients waiting to be seen. I'd groan to myself, There's got to be about 4,000 women in there, and I'm probably going to be treating at least 3,900 of them!

Most of those patients were socially and economically deprived, and many of them had sexually transmitted diseases. Human nature and my own immaturity led me to believe that only promiscuous people and those from certain socio-economic groups got "those" diseases. Later in my residency, more middle-class patients began showing up at the county hospital clinics due to rising unemployment. Also, I worked at a private hospital. This exposure to patients from differing backgrounds showed me that women from all walks of life are at risk for STDs. Yet I held on to the misconception that the women who had those diseases were different from the women I dated. I also recall prescribing medication for male and female colleagues who obviously had sexually transmitted ailments, yet I never associated my peers with the clinic patients.

My first year of transition to private practice was troublesome because I was seeing patients who'd obviously had an STD for years without knowing it. I recall telling one woman, "Ma'am, those blisters you have aren't caused by overly vigorous intercourse. You are having an outbreak of herpes, and you've had herpes for a while." She reacted with disbelief because she wanted to believe what her previous physician had told her. My guess was that her former doctor hadn't told her the truth because she was a married woman, and the chances were that she or her husband had unknowingly contracted herpes before their marriage. If you're a young gynecologist just beginning a private practice and you're $100,000 in debt, the last thing you want to do is to offend a patient. But if I hadn't told her what those blisters really were and she began having children without taking appropriate precautions, the herpes could have seriously endangered them.

Another typical patient would get angry because her general practitioner had been treating her for ten years for a "urinary tract infection," and here I was, telling her she had an STD called chlamydia. I would explain that her infection kept recurring because, being sexually transmitted, it was being passed back and forth between she and her husband. I always told the doctor involved that I was going to inform the patient, and sometimes that got me in trouble with my colleagues. But I took a stand to be loyal to my patients, even if they never came back.

> As a nurse, I'm not always present to know whether a gynecologist is telling a patient that her partner needs to be treated. I can't say they don't do it, but it's kind of funny that we don't see double prescriptions go out. We see that a doctor has prescribed seven days of Flagyl [a common treatment for trichomoniasis, a sexually transmitted vaginal infection], and that's not enough for two people. So you know that somebody's going lacking.
>
> —Joan, a nurse in a gynecological practice

I also undertook to educate my patients about STDs and to change the way they felt about themselves. Some didn't want to hear what I had to say, because they were embarrassed or ashamed. But the widespread neurosis I expected them to exhibit upon learning they had an STD did not occur. Not one threw herself out of a window! Once they were informed and had an opportunity to talk about their feelings, my patients did not feel "dirty."

The more my practice grew, the more shocked I became by the lack of information I saw among my patients. I made it a policy that patients switching to me must bring their records as a way of educating themselves. I was stunned by the number of STDs they'd unknowingly had in the past. About 40 percent of them had been treated for STDs—if you include various types of vaginitis—but the majority didn't know that their problems kept coming back because their partners weren't getting treated. They didn't know that their internal scarring from PID was caused by an untreated STD. They may have known they were having an ovary removed or a hysterectomy due to adhesions, but they didn't know that if they'd been tested ten years earlier and found to have an STD, an inexpensive dose of antibiotics could have prevented the surgery.

Early in my practice, when I started hospitalizing patients who had pelvic inflammatory disease, I was puzzled to learn that the hospital hadn't had any admissions for PID in a long time. How could that be when there were probably eighty-five gynecologists with hospital privileges? I learned that PID patients were admitted, but their surgery was coded under a different diagnosis, such as pelvic pain or belly pain. Their PID was being treated the same way I treated my own patients—I just didn't know how to play the game. The nurses on the floor used to call me the "PID king." In the doctors' lounge, the comments I'd get would be direct and to the point: "I can't believe it—are those the only patients you take care of?" One very successful doctor told me, "Eddie, I haven't seen PID in five years." I stared at him and said, "You must be blind." That was the beginning of my rebellion.

Now, I believe that doctor was sincere. In his heart, he felt he never saw PID in his patients. When it comes to sexually transmitted diseases, doctors are just as prone to denial and rationalization as their patients. For example, if a gynecologist doesn't do a culture to test his patient for chlamydia, he can say to himself, "The patient just has a pelvic infection."

> When I worked in a doctor's office, I knew that a lot of women came through with some kind of infection of their cervix. The cost to do a chlamydia culture is about the same as a course of antibiotics. So instead of

doing cultures, we usually just told the woman she had an infection and gave her antibiotics. We would tell her that her husband had to take the medicine, too, because the problem could be passed back and forth. So we gave her that hint, but the words *sexually transmitted disease* were never used. The thing is, husbands and wives don't think in terms of what gets "passed back and forth" as an STD. I didn't. Before I became a nurse, I had vaginitis, and it never occurred to me that I was giving it to my husband, and he back to me. So I don't think most patients realized that we were talking about sexual transmission.

> —Betty, a nurse in obstetrics and gynecology
> at a women's medical center

I suspect that gynecologists begin to pick up a sort of indirect dishonesty during internships and residencies, when they are primarily treating low-income patients in county hospital clinics. Some of those patients have never had a private physician. They come in one time and might never come in again, so the doctor-patient relationship has little chance to develop. When a resident has been up all night and a woman is brought in dying from a tubal pregnancy, he doesn't have the time to explain to her that the source of her problem is PID, let alone that it is sexually transmitted. But clinic patients who aren't in critical condition may not get much more attention from a busy resident.

> Do you know which patients doctors are most likely to inform about having an STD? They are indigent patients. A doctor will roll in and tell an indigent patient in plain English, "You've got the clap." He's not going to get compensated for taking care of her, and he's not worried about losing her as a patient or hurting her feelings.
>
> —Ann, a nurse at a teaching hospital

Most gynecologists don't face that kind of clientele once they enter private practice. Yet some still don't initiate discussions on sexual transmission of disease, simply because they don't want to take the time or the responsibility to educate their patients. They're too busy and successful. The irony is that STDs are a huge source of revenue for these doctors. They may rationalize that they can help more people if they don't spend a lot of time with individual patients. But the bottom line for these doctors is just that— the bottom line. If they spent more time answering questions and educating their patients, they couldn't see as many paying customers in a day.

> Some doctors are just unwilling to take the time to answer questions. There are exceptions, but from what I've seen, the average amount of time a gynecologist spends just talking with a patient is less than five minutes.
> —Shelly, a floor nurse on an ob/gyn ward

Furthermore, as a rule, we don't begin our practices having a lot of social skills. During the past two decades, the selection process to get into medical school hasn't exactly favored the Marcus Welby type of candidate. Preparation for medical school requires almost constant study. Either we marry during medical school, or we spend the long years of training virtually married to our schooling, with very little time to date or even interact with anyone outside of the medical profession. So we tend to start our practices with a social deficit when it comes to interpersonal relationships. That is one reason a patient may say, "He's a good doctor but he just doesn't talk to me."

Another reason gynecologists may not discuss the sexually transmitted nature of their patients' problems is that we just don't know how to talk about it. Our medical training gives us the technical information we need, but most of us didn't have any training—either in medical school or afterward—in human sexuality or how to discuss sensitive issues with patients. Some training programs are beginning to incorporate role-playing, but they are still the exception. When we get into private practice and a patient's lifestyle and emotions are involved with the problem she is bringing to us, we may not know how to deal with that.

> I've observed that a lot of doctors can't even look a woman in the eye and talk to her. They're people, and they have the same hang-ups that the rest of us do.
>
> —Carlotta, a registered nurse

I learned that if your doctor isn't equipped, or willing, or up front enough to talk about sex, you've got a problem. I was having a recurring problem with genital warts. I didn't know what they were, so I saw my doctor. Basically, his response was, 'I'll give you some pills. Take them and come back in thirty days.' A month later everything was gone. When I saw him a year later, he said, 'You've got a little something. Let's give you some antibiotics and I'll see you in thirty days.' Again, a month later everything looked fine. Next year, things still looked okay. The fourth year, there it was again.

He talked superficially with me, then recommended a biopsy. I trusted that he was taking good care of me, so I made an appointment. Mind you, all this time my husband never entered the equation. I had asked once whether the doctor should check my husband. He answered that if there was a problem with my husband, I'd see it.

I met another gynecologist as a business acquaintance shortly before I was to undergo a colposcopy [a procedure in which a special magnifying instrument is used to examine the vagina and cervix]. I found myself telling him about my recurring problem. He asked me what my Pap smear had indicated, but I didn't know. I'd never seen the report. He said to me, 'You're an intelligent woman, and you've never seen your Pap test?' He also suggested that my husband be checked by a doctor.

When I requested my records, my doctor apparently interpreted the request to mean that I questioned his judgment. It took weeks for him to get a copy of my records to me. When he finally did, he enclosed a condescending letter, which said in part: 'You're an intelligent woman, and I trust that you understand that on a scale of one to ten, this is a little thing, and I would tell you if it were a bigger thing.' When the warts first showed up they may have been a minor thing, but long-term? Maybe not so minor.

Well, my husband got himself to a doctor and, sure enough, he had the warts. We'd been passing them back and forth. Once we knew that, we were able to control the problem, in about a month, what we'd been batting around for four years—all because my doctor wasn't willing to talk about sex.

—Selina, a 37-year-old executive secretary

Sometimes the problem goes even deeper. Doctors are human beings, and we are not immune to narrow-minded attitudes. As people, most of us have had as hard a time as the rest of society adjusting to the sexual revolution of the past few decades. In fact, I feel that as professionals, doctors are ten to fifteen years behind the rest of society in accepting changes in lifestyle.

One such doctor occasionally calls me to make a referral saying, "Listen, I don't want to take care of this woman. She sleeps with two guys, and I can't deal with her." I knew another gynecologist on the staff of a hospital that had a good cross-section of conservative and liberal physicians.

He used to refer patients to me whom he did not want in his practice, calling them "fornicators." He gave them that label simply because they'd had sex before getting married. He is an extreme example, I'll grant you, but that doctor affects the lives of a lot of women in the city where he practices.

The point is that there is no room for a narrow-minded or judgmental attitude in medicine. Since gynecology deals with the health of the reproductive organs, and your sexual practices have so much to do with your health in that area, both you and your gynecologist must feel comfortable talking about your sex life.

There are gynecologists out there—even the younger ones—who skirt the issue of STDs because they can't bring themselves to ask their patients about their sexual lifestyles. I'll give you an example. In my capacity as coordinator of a hospital's residency training program in gynecology, I encounter young doctors who find it an unimaginable perversion that some people practice anal sex. Now, I'm not saying that doctors have to like anal sex in their personal lives, but anal sex is a risk factor for many sexually transmitted diseases, such as hepatitis B and AIDS. As professionals, doctors who can't bring themselves to ask about sexual practices like these can't effectively screen their patients for exposure to STDs.

Some doctors assume that if they tell a woman some unpleasant facts, she is likely to have a breakdown. Today, doctors take it for granted that women are intelligent and capable—except when they come to the gynecologist's office. Certainly, it's natural for a woman to feel upset at being diagnosed with an STD. When I give a patient news like that, she may cry, but life goes on, and we work together to solve the problem. A woman's displeasure at being diagnosed with an STD is nothing compared to the anger she feels when she learns that she is infertile or has invasive

cervical cancer because she wasn't told she had an STD back
when that knowledge could have done her some good.

> Some doctors just rationalize that it's in the patient's
> best interest not to know. They don't want to hurt her
> feelings. But when a patient doesn't know what's hap-
> pening to her, sometimes she becomes that hypochon-
> driac, or that neurotic "witch" that I've heard doctors
> label nervous, frightened patients. Maybe if her doctor
> told her she had an STD she would say, "Thank God!
> Now I can live with it. At least I have something real,
> and I know what it is."
>
> —Delores, a nurse in a group practice
>   of gynecologists

A patient's marital status should make no difference as to
how much her gynecologist tells her about her condition.
But when a married patient is diagnosed with an STD, a
gynecologist can be uncomfortable enough to hide the fact.

> I think doctors are afraid of instigating conflict be-
> tween the partners. Let's say you're dealing with infer-
> tility, so you've got a couple who are already under a
> lot of stress about their sexuality. When you can rem-
> edy their situation with antibiotics, would you want to
> interject conflict by bringing up something that might
> point to an extramarital affair? I think we do have an
> obligation as medical people to inform our patients.
> But when you're talking about being a medical person
> on the one side, and a human being on the other, it's
> hard to get on that fence post.
>
> —Deanna, a resident in obstetrics and
>   gynecology

Believe me, I do not relish this conflict. But let's say this
couple's infertility was the result of an extramarital affair that

brought chlamydia into the relationship. If I didn't inform them and the affairs continued, their medical treatment would do no good; if they went on to have a child, it might be born with conjunctivitis (an eye inflammation) or more serious problems.

There is no room for debate here. Our job as physicians is to tell our patients all of the facts about their disease and its treatment. We have to be diplomatic, and it can be difficult to discuss the intimate details of a couple's relationship. But if I have to remove your uterus and ovaries and you're twenty-five years old, how much more intimate can I get?

As we've discussed, pelvic pain or infection, pain during intercourse, PID, ectopic or tubal pregnancy, infertility, abnormal Pap smears, precancerous cervical cells, and cervical cancer (not to mention procedures such as laparoscopy, laser surgery, cone biopsy, cryosurgery, laparotomy, hysterectomy, and in vitro fertilization) are all things you may have heard about without knowing enough to make the connection that these were probably related to a sexually transmitted disease.

If not being told that you have an STD can cause such devastating results, you may be wondering if you have any legal right to that information. Why don't women simply take these doctors to court? Why aren't there so many legal cases that gynecologists sit up and take notice—start leveling with patients? Although I am not a lawyer and a comprehensive discussion of legal issues is beyond the scope of this book, I think this is a reasonable question and worthy of further discussion.

There is a legal principle called the doctrine of informed consent, which would seem to apply to this issue. All the states recognize some form of this doctrine, although each jurisdiction has its own interpretation. The premise of informed consent is that a patient has the right to make decisions concerning proposed medical treatment. Informed consent generally means that before a doctor subjects a patient to any risky procedures, he must disclose to the patient: the diagnosis; a description of the proposed treatment and its purpose; the outcome the doctor expects and the probability of success; the risks, benefits, and consequences of the treatment; information about alternatives to the proposed treatment; and the effect of no treatment or procedure being performed, including the prognosis and risks associated with no treatment.

Case by case, the informed consent doctrine is evolving. Although the standards that are used to measure a physician's duty to inform the patient vary, the trend is for courts to assess a doctor's duty to disclose based on the information that the average, reasonable patient would need in order to make an intelligent choice. If you would like to find out how cases involving informed consent have fared in the jurisdiction in which you live, most law school libraries subscribe to computerized search networks that can provide this information on a case-by-case or a legal precedent basis. If a doctor's failure to inform you about your medical condition has resulted in your having to undergo procedures you would not have needed otherwise, or has resulted in your developing health problems, it is well within your rights to consult a lawyer.

Realistically, you should know that applying the informed consent doctrine to the issue of STDs isn't as simple as it sounds. Few legal cases are on record involving informed consent and STDs. One probable reason is that most of these cases are settled out of court. Furthermore, until more women understand the consequences of STDs, many women who have grounds for a case will not turn to the legal system for help.

The legal system can become a major ally for women who are victimized by being kept in the dark about STDs.

However, before this can happen, the public will have to become aware of the direct causal link between STDs and serious medical problems. The problem is, most damage caused by STDs is discovered years after a woman first contracted the disease.

One challenge here is that an illness such as cervical cancer can involve so many variables that the patient may not realize she was not fully informed a few years earlier. By the time abnormal cervical cells have progressed into cervical cancer with noticeable symptoms, a woman may no longer be seeing the doctor who was treating her when she first began having abnormal Pap smears. For example, a doctor at a university health clinic may have treated a college-age patient for a "pelvic infection"; where will that doctor be five or ten years later, when this woman finds she is unable to bear children because that "infection"—which was actually PID as a result of chlamydia or gonorrhea—has been causing a buildup of scar tissue inside her all those years?

Tina, now in her mid-twenties, is a case in point. She had an upper-middle-class upbringing and began having sex at seventeen. Within that first year, Tina contracted such a severe case of PID that she had to be hospitalized. A culture performed at the time tested positive for gonorrhea, but neither Tina nor her parents were informed. "I didn't ask how I got the infection because at that age, I didn't know how to question a doctor. To a young person, a doctor is somebody whom you trust, you respect," says Tina. Also, because nobody told Tina that she'd had an STD, she didn't know that her partner needed to be treated.

After Tina left the hospital, she continued to experience pelvic pain. "I saw five or six doctors, and everyone said it was in my head," she recalls. "They gave me pain pills and antibiotics, but when the pain didn't go away, they told my parents that I was a hypochondriac." Tina subsequently had another severe PID infection and had to be hospitalized for ten days.

This time the doctors told Tina and her parents what had caused her PID, but the damage was already done. She had lost about 30 percent of her fertility to extensive scarring and began suffering chronic pain. After Tina married, she underwent surgery to unblock her fallopian tubes. She has been able to have one child, but a second tubal surgery (which was not covered by insurance) was unsuccessful, and she is now infertile. She will probably need a hysterectomy to relieve her pain.

Tina is understandably angry. If the doctor who treated her during her first hospitalization had informed her about having an STD, Tina—who was monogamous—would have seen that her partner went for treatment. That could have prevented her second hospitalization, and the problems her PID still causes her today.

Aside from doctors who deliberately keep their patients in the dark about having an STD, there is another way patients go uninformed. The good news about the scenario I'm going to describe is that you can do something to prevent it.

Beverly went to her long-time gynecologist for a Pap smear and got a phone call from her doctor's office saying the results were negative, or normal. Her Pap smears had always been normal, so it was eighteen months later when Beverly came in for her next Pap. (At that time, the guidelines of the American Cancer Society stated that if a woman had three consecutive normal Paps, she only needed a Pap smear every three years. As we'll discuss in Chapter 4, I feel that a sexually active woman should have a pelvic exam and Pap smear every year.)

That second Pap smear, Beverly was shocked to discover, showed her with early cervical cancer. How had cancer developed so quickly and without warning? It hadn't. The pathologist who filled out her Pap smear report eighteen months earlier had made a notation that Beverly had abnormal cells, but he had checked the wrong box, indicating incorrectly that hers was a Class I smear, meaning she showed no atypical changes. Beverly's Pap smear report clearly showed a contradiction, but her doctor never personally checked Pap reports unless they were labeled Class II or higher. Compounding these two errors, Beverly's report was misfiled by a clerk in the doctor's office.

Initially, Beverly's only question was why she now had cancer after being normal only eighteen months earlier. When her doctor ignored her reasonable requests for an explanation, Beverly filed suit. "If my doctor had returned my calls, even once, and talked to me, there's no way I would have initiated a lawsuit," says Beverly. "People who know me are amazed I did that, because I'm just not that way."

Beverly's case was settled out of court. Although she was in the right and received financial compensation, Beverly paid a high price, too. She had to undergo a cone biopsy in the hospital (see Chapter 4), which is not an innocuous procedure. One of the risks involved is cervical stenosis in which the cervical canal becomes blocked, preventing fertility.

Also, Beverly's medical insurance was canceled. This would not have happened if her problem had been detected at the precancerous stage. But now she bears the label "cancer patient," and no insurance company will carry her.

What can you learn from Beverly's story? Errors can happen every day. Laboratories can check the wrong box on a Pap smear result. The doctor you've trusted for years can hire a clerk who mislabels or misfiles your test results. If your name is Sally M. Jones, your doctor's office might call you and read you the Pap test results for Sally N. Jones. You can end up not knowing you have an STD, or worse, not knowing you have developed a serious medical problem.

The kind of patient you are also affects the extent to which your doctor is able to inform you. Some patients really don't want to know the truth. They don't ask any questions and they don't let their gynecologists know when they haven't understood what he has told them.

Some women don't put themselves in a position to be informed. For instance, many women don't go to the doctor when they experience pelvic pain or pain during intercourse. I see patients all the time who accept pain without asking themselves about its cause. Some women are embarrassed to tell their doctors when they experience pain during intercourse (which is not normal and should never be ignored).

Furthermore, old attitudes about venereal diseases die hard. Some women feel so shamed and guilty at the prospect of having an STD that they never give their gynecologist a chance to help them.

> I had a perfectly fine gynecologist. For more than ten years I felt I was in the best of hands. But when I suspected I might have caught something from having sex, I didn't feel I could go to my own doctor. Sometimes there are certain people that you don't feel you can discuss certain things with. You have to have a certain rapport. It's not that I couldn't have gotten good help had I approached him with what I was worried about, but I never tried. I felt he might judge me, so I went to a clinic instead so nobody would know who I was. I didn't want anybody to be able to look at my records. I just wanted to be anonymous Patient X.
>
> —Angela, a bank teller

You have a right, as a patient, to tell your doctor anything. Sometimes opening up may feel like a gamble. From what my patients tell me, they are initially embarrassed to ask me to test them for STDs. But once they see that I'm not going to judge them, they want to be tested for everything. If your own doctor doesn't respond adequately, you can and should change doctors.

Earlier we talked about the harm doctors do when they deliberately don't tell patients they have an STD-related problem. Even if your doctor only makes a mistake—as in Beverly's case—the outcome is the same. The solution is the same, too.

If your doctor says you have a medical problem, get the right information. Every abnormality has a cause, so don't accept the explanation that "it just got there" or those abnormal cells "just happened." If your doctor knows enough about the problem to prescribe a method of treatment, then he must know the cause. If the cause is an STD, then that is vital information you need to know in order to get the proper treatment and to prevent serious problems down the line.

Always obtain a copy of the actual lab report on your Pap smear. Tell your doctor to put a note in your file saying that every Pap test report should be mailed to you. That report is yours; you paid for it. You can easily learn enough about Pap test reports to catch the kind of mistake Beverly's pathologist made (see Chapter 4). You can learn to recognize when your report indicates a problem, and know the nature of that problem. It is not hard. It is your responsibility as a patient.

Now, I know you may have to embolden yourself and get past your shyness or embarrassment simply to ask the right questions, but your responsibility doesn't end with asking questions. Don't accept just any answer that you get. Ask yourself, Did my doctor's response really answer my question to my satisfaction? It's important to know when you are not getting an answer that is accurate. Make sure you get your questions answered, but remember that your doctor may have some very human reasons for finding it difficult to talk to you. Approach him not on a confrontational level, but on a human level.

I know you want to put all your trust in your doctor. You may have had the same doctor for many years, and you may like him or her very much. But doctors are human.

They make clerical mistakes, and they make mistakes in judgment. Mistakes don't matter in a lot of other professions, but when it comes to the medical profession, you can't afford to leave total responsibility for your health in the hands of any one person, no matter how much you look up to them. There must be not one—but two—people looking out for your interests, checking and double-checking your Pap test results, and asking vital questions about your care. It's time to become a partner with your doctor. The next chapter will tell you how.

PART TWO

CHAPTER 3

Rx: Becoming Partners with Your Gynecologist

How to get the answers you need and the care you deserve

When I was a young intern in obstetrics and gynecology, I treated a lot of hospital clinic patients, as most interns do. Like many of my peers, I began to fall into the trap of seeing myself as an "almighty provider." One day a patient, who was waiting for a gynecological exam, tried to tell me she was uncomfortable. I made an insensitive reply, something to the effect that a pelvic exam was no big deal.

What happened next changed the course of my career, thanks to a remarkable man, Dr. Pelham Staples, who was both my mentor and the chief of the hospital's training programs for interns and residents in obstetrics and gynecology.

Overhearing my remark, Dr. Staples said we were going to pretend that I was the patient to whom I had just been rude. He sent me into an examining room and had a nurse tell me to get undressed and put on one of those flimsy little gowns. He must have set the thermostat at thirty-five degrees; then he kept me waiting by myself for what seemed an hour. Finally, he came in with the nurse and asked me perfunctorily if I had any questions. With my rear exposed and my masculinity in shambles, the last thing I wanted to do was ask questions. Next he told me to put my feet in the stirrups. I didn't know Dr. Staples very well, and I thought he must be crazy. He put gloves on and spread my legs—and I knew he was crazy. He touched my bottom with a speculum that felt as though it had been chilled to forty degrees below zero. Then he got up and said, "Young man, don't you ever make a patient feel the way you do right now. Don't you ever forget this." And I never did.

From that day on, I never again regarded patients as merely bodies to examine; I knew they had feelings. I'd had a taste of the embarrassment women feel at the gynecologist's office. I now understood that simply telling women to relax is nonsense. No woman in her right mind is going to relax in a gynecologist's office, especially if she expects an impersonal and demeaning experience. I resolved to make patients feel respected, and to treat them with kindness and sensitivity—the same would apply if I were a urologist taking care of male patients.

If you were to ask me today how to choose a good gynecologist (or a good physician in any area of medicine), I would say that kindness and a respectful manner are essential. In fact, I'd suggest that instead of looking for a good gynecologist, you look for a good *relationship* with a gynecologist. There is a difference.

Let's say you found a kind, respectful gynecologist with impressive credentials. Would he be the best gynecologist for you? That depends. Would you feel comfortable telling him what he would need to know about your sexual activities or asking him about any sexual problems you might have? If you thought you had contracted a sexually transmitted disease (STD), could you, without hesitation, go to him to be checked? Could you count on him to inform you if he diagnosed an STD? Would he encourage you to ask questions? Would he take the time to bring up the questions you didn't think of or were embarrassed to ask? Would he educate you and make sure you understood his explanations?

What I have been describing is a doctor-patient partnership. There's a rationale for this that goes way beyond making the patient's experience more pleasant just because that's the decent thing to do. Gynecologists must step down from the pedestals they and their patients have placed them on, and deal with their patients as respected partners, in order to facilitate an important aspect of doctor-patient communication.

The experiences individual women shared in earlier chapters confirm that it is vital that gynecologists communicate with patients about their findings, but the need for communication is actually much broader. If we back up and look at how doctors reach those findings, we'd learn that it's rare when a doctor is able to make a diagnosis based on physical evidence alone. Even though gynecologists have a lot of fancy tests and equipment at their disposal, a doctor isn't going to know which test to order or what diagnostic procedure to perform unless he and his patient communicate. However, communication is useless unless both parties—gynecologist and patient—do their part. Both have vital information to convey, and both must be good listeners.

> When I went for my annual exam and my gynecologist asked if I had anything to report, I said I was fine. Actually, I was embarrassed to mention that every time my husband penetrated deeply during intercourse, it was very painful. I was only a little uncomfortable during the examination, so I wasn't going to say anything. But my doctor asked if there were any problems I had forgotten to mention. So I took a deep breath and told him what was happening with me. He also asked if my husband had any symptoms, and when I checked, I found out my husband had some burning

with urination and a discharge he hadn't told me
about. I'm glad I talked freely with my doctor. That led
him to do some tests, and he was able to treat some
pelvic scarring I had before it got to the point where
I became infertile or needed a hysterectomy.

　　　—Liz, a housewife

Open, honest communication can't take place in a setting
where either party feels uncomfortable, inhibited, inferior,
or judged. That's why the relationship between you and
your gynecologist must be a partnership, a collaboration.

What would such a partnership be like? To give you a
feel for what I'm talking about, imagine you're making your
first office visit to a new gynecologist for a routine checkup
and gynecological exam. First you visit Dr. A.

You arrive a few minutes early to find that Dr. A is running way behind due to an emergency; his staff never
bothered to phone you to reschedule. When you ask the
receptionist how long you will have to wait, she is discour-
teous and unhelpful. Finally, a bored-looking nurse has you
provide a urine sample, then conducts you to an examination room, tells you to undress and put on a skimpy gown,
does a few tests, and leaves you alone. You wait. There are
no magazines to read and you have goosebumps rising all
over you. You seem to wait forever.

Eventually, Dr. A comes in, rushes through a few questions without giving you a chance to ask any of your own,
and has you put your feet in the stirrups. Without any explanation he inserts—not very gently—what feels like an ice-
cold speculum. When you reflexively tighten every muscle
in your pelvis, he says, "Honey, relax. It's no big deal."

When the examination is over, Dr. A heads quickly
for the door. "If you don't have any questions, we'll let
you know the results," he says and is gone before you can
even blink.

Once you are dressed, the nurse conducts you to the receptionist's desk, where a bill is handed to you without explanation. The charges are higher than you were previously quoted for an office visit, and when you question them, the receptionist curtly tells you they are lab fees for extra cultures. You tell her you don't know what these cultures were for, and you ask to speak to Dr. A; she simply replies, "Dr. A is with another patient. He'll send you the results." You never get a chance to go over your exam or Dr. A's findings.

In a week or two, you get a form letter from Dr. A's office telling you your Pap test results were normal or abnormal, nothing more. Worse yet, this announcement comes on a postcard, so you can be sure that your mail carrier is as informed as you are! If your results were abnormal, the worst-case scenario is that the notice arrives on a Friday, and when—in a panic—you try to reach Dr. A, his office informs you he is gone for the weekend. You spend the longest, most frightening weekend of your life waiting until you can call him on Monday.

Perhaps the notice says that your results were normal, but you want to ask Dr. A some questions about medication or other concerns. When you call, the nurse won't put you through to him. She says she will find out the responses to your questions, but you never get what feel like satisfactory answers. You ask her to have Dr. A call you when he has time, but you never hear from him. Have you come to expect the kind of treatment provided by our imaginary Dr. A?

Now imagine, instead, that you are calling Dr. B for an appointment. The receptionist pleasantly and courteously tells you how much time to allocate for your visit and takes your phone number so she can inform you of any major delays. Not long after you arrive, Dr. B greets you and ushers you into the privacy of his office. You chat for a few minutes, getting to know one another, and then he asks all the questions necessary for him to gain a thorough understanding of your needs (Chapter 4 will cover the gyneco-logical exam and Pap smear in detail.). He also encourages you to ask questions. He explains the procedures he is going to perform during the exam and tells you he will let you know if he needs to run any additional tests.

When you feel satisfied that you have no more questions, a nurse conducts you to an examining room, leaves while you undress and don an examining gown, then returns to do her tests. She leaves you with some reading material, but it is not long before she or another woman in the role of chaperone returns with Dr. B. In addition to assisting him, she will serve as a third set of ears to pass on any informa-tion you may need about your exam in the future, should Dr. B be unable to speak to you.

Dr. B is gentle and considerate during the examination, explaining each step of the procedure beforehand and how it will feel. He encourages you to ask questions as they come up. He does the little things that add to your comfort, such as warming the speculum, and uses extra lubrication or a smaller speculum if you are too uncomfortable. If Dr. B sees a need to perform tests not covered under the rou-tine examination, he explains the tests and additional costs.

After the exam is over and you are dressed, Dr. B invites you back to his office to discuss the findings of your exam. He explains anything you don't understand and encourages you to tell him or ask him anything you may have forgotten during the examination. He also spells out when and how you will receive your test results, as well as pertinent office policies.

Your test results come to you in the form of a phone call or a letter from Dr. B. In the event of an abnormal finding, Dr. B—not a nurse—calls to notify you and discuss your options. He also provides you with a copy of your Pap test lab report and explains what it means.

Have you already concluded that you would rather have Dr. B for your gynecologist? What about Dr. B makes him

your choice? More to the point, what is it about Dr. B that
makes him the better candidate for a doctor-patient partnership? Being his patient would be a more pleasant experience, but there's more to it than that. Everything about Dr.
B and his practice creates an environment in which you can
relate to one another as collaborators in your health care.
Relating as partners makes it more likely that you will feel
able to speak freely about topics you find sensitive or
embarrassing, and ask questions without fearing that they
will be considered silly or ignorant. As though you were
trusted business partners, you and your gynecologist will
expect no less than a full exchange of questions and information from one another. That is the straight talk to which
the title of this book refers, the kind of communication that
could save your life.

How can you have this type of relationship with a gynecologist? There *are* physicians like Dr. B, but you may have
to hunt to find them. While the partnership approach has
begun to catch on in specialties such as family practice and
pediatrics, gynecology is primarily taught as a traditional
surgical specialty. Medical schools and the advanced training programs that educate gynecologists don't customarily
teach courses on how to relate to patients as partners. In
fact, very few medical curriculums include courses on communicating with patients. While other service-oriented
occupations have a pretty good track record in providing
customer-service training, gynecologists must develop
people skills on their own.

Medicine is, however, a business as well as an art, and
businesses must eventually respond to consumer demand
or fail to compete in the marketplace. When you see a
gynecologist, you are a consumer purchasing a service. In
this chapter, and throughout the rest of this book, my aim
is to empower you to make informed choices for your own
care and to create change by putting consumer demand to

work. Once you know that a doctor-patient partnership is possible, I hope you will encourage it, demand it, and help build the practices of those gynecologists who offer it.

As I see it, the way I can empower you to create the best possible relationship with your gynecologist is to help you get a feel for what that relationship should be like. Our imaginary Dr. B has already provided a sketch of that relationship in action. Now let's flesh out some of the blank areas, starting with the way your gynecologist should interact with you, and how you can best interact with him.

One suggestion before we go on: As this doctor-patient partnership becomes clearer in your mind, you might want to think about what you want out of your relationship with a gynecologist. In your opinion, what are your rights and responsibilities as a patient, and what rights and responsibilities does your doctor have?

How does a good gynecologist interact with you?

First impressions are important, and your first chance to gain a feel for your gynecologist—during the initial visit and every visit thereafter—will be your interaction with his office staff. If you have a problem with his staff, then you may have a problem with your doctor; after all, he hired them and he is ultimately in charge of managing them. The way a good doctor interacts with you begins with the way his staff interacts with you. A professional staff handles the scheduling of appointments as any well-run business would, respecting the value of your time. They are helpful when you need an explanation about a bill or assistance with paperwork, and it goes without saying that they are courteous and pleasant.

When a patient isn't pleasant and courteous, a good gynecologist, as well as his office staff, understand that something may be wrong. For example, my receptionist once mentioned that the patient waiting to see me, a woman in her early twenties, seemed to be in a terrible mood. When I examined her, she was extremely rude and abrupt. However, the reason soon became clear. She had a ruptured tubal pregnancy; she was hemorrhaging and near death. We rushed her to the hospital, and after emergency surgery, she recovered. When she came to my office for her follow-up visit, she was a very sweet person. Not only did she not remember how rude she had been, she didn't even remember being in my office. She had been in shock. From that day on, my office personnel understood that a difficult patient might be a sick patient.

I'm not the friendliest patient at the dentist's office, so I understand that patients react differently in stressful situations. Some patients tell offensive jokes, some giggle, some get clammy hands. A good doctor is understanding, so there is no need for you to be embarrassed by how you act under pressure. If your doctor finds your actions as a patient inappropriate, he will tell you. If he doesn't want to take care of you, he will send you a letter telling you that. But until you get that letter, you have every right to be cared for in a proper, professional way.

What if, when you call your gynecologist with questions, you can only get through to a nurse? If you feel that you are getting satisfactory information, having a nurse take your calls is acceptable. But don't hesitate to ask if the nurse spoke to the doctor. And if you truly feel that you should talk to the doctor, insist on that, because his expertise is the service you are paying for.

This brings up what is probably the most important factor that sets apart the kind of doctor who should be your partner in health care. A good gynecologist believes his role is to educate patients, not only about what is wrong with them, but about how to prevent health problems in the first place. He doesn't see educating patients as a burden; he doesn't mind that once you become better informed, you will be able to ask more questions and, thus, take up more of his time. Rather than have you stay an uninformed, passive recipient of health care, he understands that the more you know, the easier you will ultimately make his job and the better you can participate in safeguarding your own health.

Sadly, the trend today is toward educational video rooms in every gynecologist's office. I don't have a patient education room; I'm getting paid to educate my patients. Having a patient watch videos saves a little of the doctor's time, but it doesn't teach that patient to ask questions, and it doesn't help doctor or patient to become comfortable communicating with each other. When I am explaining something to a patient and a visual aid is needed, I often do drawings on the spot. No matter how serious her condition is, she enjoys a little humor laughing at my artwork. More importantly, we communicate one-on-one at her pace until she understands my explanation. Since she is an active participant, she remembers my unartistic scribbling better than she would retain any memory of a video.

The more questions you ask, the more opportunities you give your doctor to serve as an educator. A good doctor understands that the average patient may not know what to ask and feel intimidated as a result. He will encourage and prompt you so that you develop the skill of forming questions or asking for clarification of explanations. If he sees that you are apprehensive or embarrassed to ask questions about sex, he will help you talk about your sexuality as it relates to your health.

As we saw with Liz, above, a good doctor is as much a listener as he is an educator. Apparently, listening is becoming a lost art among physicians. One study published in a recent issue of the Journal of the American Medical Association timed how long patients were able to talk before their doctors interrupted them. The average doctor interrupted his patient after only eighteen seconds!

Some of the sexually transmitted diseases we'll be discussing later in this book are hard for a physician to spot through visual examination alone. Diagnosis often depends on the simplest, most innocuous-sounding statements made by a patient. A good gynecologist will draw you out, encouraging you to tell him anything that might fill in his picture of your medical history and lifestyle or give him a clue regarding your medical condition.

It should go without saying that this gynecologist will take you seriously when you tell him what you think is wrong. He won't tell you that a problem you're having is "in your head," at least not before doing everything possible to rule out a physical cause, but that is exactly what happened to one patient who seemed to have everything going for her. She was a nurse on the gynecological floor of a major hospital, and she had a female gynecologist.

> I work side by side with Dr. X and went to her for my annual checkups. She even delivered my children. I never had any illnesses or complaints. So when I went in for the first time with a list of problems, I had every expectation that Dr. X would try to find out what was wrong. But she didn't listen to me. She commented that I was getting older and wasn't on the pill anymore, then tried to tell me that I was in pain because I was ovulating. You don't have to be an ob/gyn nurse to know that you don't ovulate on the ninth day of your cycle! I insisted on having a sonogram, and the radiologist told me it looked like I had a hemorrhagic cyst, meaning a cyst bleeding into itself. When I called Dr. X the next day, she said, 'We'll probably watch you for a month and then repeat the sonogram, but the results aren't back yet, so call me tomorrow.' When I called the next day, and then the day after that, I was

never able to speak to the doctor. 'Take it easy for a month,' the nurse told me, so I asked her what that meant. Could I pick up my toddler? Could I have sex with my husband? 'I'll ask and get back to you,' she promised, but she never did.

I knew I needed to see another doctor, but it was hard emotionally, because this was someone I'd entrusted my body and my care to for eight years. The doctor that I switched to tells me that when he phoned Dr. X, she told him that I was crazy and neurotic. Well, it turned out that I had such extensive endometriosis that I needed a hysterectomy. To this day, Dr. X and I still see each other every day at the same hospital, and she won't even say hello or make eye contact with me.

—Carol, a hospital nurse

As we discussed in Chapter 2, a gynecologist-partner won't dismiss your problem as "just a little virus," "just a little bacteria," or something that "just happens." Every abnormality has a cause. He'll be honest with you and educate you about the problem, so you are informed enough to cooperate in your treatment. He'll see that your partner is treated in the case of a sexually transmitted disease, and that you do all you can in the way of prevention.

One of my female colleagues (a gynecologist in the Pacific Northwest) sums up the issue of communication between women and their doctors very clearly. "Women are discounted," she says. "Our complaints are discounted and our sense about our own bodies is discounted, but our assessment of our own symptoms is usually right on. We're good at that. Women want medical care in an atmosphere where somebody's going to listen, where somebody's going to validate what they're feeling. A lot of that isn't science; a lot of that is art. It is making eye contact, listening, telling the patient she isn't crazy, and agreeing to find the problem and get it under control. Once you've done that, a patient can relax, and as she talks, a lot of other things will come out that may help to explain her condition."

How can you best interact with your gynecologist?

Just as your gynecologist is a professional with a job to perform, you too have a job to perform, one that is vital to the quality of care you receive. It is your job—and your right—to ask questions, to make sure those questions get answered, and to provide all the information that your gynecologist needs to do his job. It is your responsibility to interact with your doctor in whatever way facilitates your ability to hold up your end of the relationship.

A good example of what I mean by facilitating communication is the matter of your being dressed or undressed in your doctor's presence. It is only natural to feel intimidated, embarrassed, or distracted when you are undressed in the presence of a person with whom you are not on mutually intimate terms. The only proper time for you to be undressed in your gynecologist's presence is during the examination. When the two of you are exchanging information and making decisions about your health care, everything about your interaction and the setting you are in has to be conducive to concentration and communication. You have enough to deal with, having to digest complicated information in a situation most people find stressful, let alone having a medical problem that may upset you. So make things easy on yourself: insist that your gynecologist extend you the courtesy of talking to you in a private setting while you are dressed. This is not an option, but a matter of ethical conduct between physician and patient.

I never meet a patient for the first time in the examining room with her clothes off. You have to meet patients as people. If both of you are dressed, you can have eye contact. Patients tell me more when they are dressed, and they remember more of what we discuss.

—Lilly, a gynecologist

If a gynecologist won't talk to you before he examines you, that's demeaning. I look at that as a power play by the doctor to establish who's in control of the situation. When you're the one who's sitting there with the little sheet wrapped around you, and they're standing there looking down at you, you're not in control.

If a doctor won't take the time to talk to you and answer your questions before he examines you, you don't need to be there.

—Adele, a gynecological nurse

It is also your right to have your partner, another family member, or a friend present when you and your doctor are discussing your care. As the saying goes, sometimes two pairs of ears are better than one. This person may remember to ask any questions you forget to raise. Since they are in a better position than you are to be objective and aren't under the stress of being a patient, they can help you remember afterward what your gynecologist said. You can always ask them to leave the room if the discussion gets into any areas you wish kept private.

You should be able to talk to your gynecologist about anything. If you break up with your partner because he was sleeping with someone else, we need to know that, because you might have contracted an STD. If your husband is having an affair, we need to know, because he could be infected with HIV. If you develop a problem related to sex (such as painful intercourse), we need to know that because it could be a symptom of a serious illness (such as endometriosis or pelvic inflammatory disease). Don't be embarrassed to discuss your personal problems with us. If we feel we cannot handle all of that responsibility, we will refer you to a counselor or therapist.

Remember that you are there to ask and to understand. No doubt you routinely ask questions of other service providers—if you go to a hair stylist, you probably ask all kinds of questions before you let anyone cut or perm your hair. But many women coming to a gynecologist are so intimidated that they don't ask questions. Would you hesitate to talk to your auto mechanic about a problem you're having with your brakes, knowing that every time you get in your car you could be risking serious injury or death? The consequences of not communicating well with your gynecologist can be just as lethal.

Believe me, to the right gynecologist there is no such thing as a silly or dumb question. The only dumb question is the one that was never asked. An operating room nurse told me once that as she was prepping a patient for a hysterectomy, the woman asked her, "Nurse, how soon after the operation will I be able to have children?" Now, there's a question that should have been asked a bit earlier—back at her doctor's office!

If you come home from the doctor's office and think of questions you forgot to ask, call him. A good doctor will not be upset because you did.

Unless you are a physician yourself, there are bound to be times when you don't understand your doctor's explanations. Let him know, and help him clarify things for you, perhaps by rephrasing your question or by asking him to show you a picture or model that would make his description clearer. Whether the topic is the reproductive anatomy you may not have studied since high school or a surgical procedure you need, the gynecologist who wants to be your partner in health care will be happy to explain things until you understand them.

The kind of explanations I usually get from doctors are very general, and I think that's why questions don't come up. I'm not saying they whitewash anything, but if a doctor only gives you the overall picture, and doesn't touch on the details, you don't feel that it's anything you need to be concerned about.
—Kay, a teacher

Before we leave the topic of partnership interaction between gynecologist and patient, I want to raise the issue of touch as an expression of support and affection. In some quarters, hugging a patient or holding her hand before surgery or when she is nervous in the examining room is seen to have sexual connotations. I'll never forget the day I attended a medical symposium, and the guest lecturer said that it was only acceptable to sit next to a hospitalized patient and hold her hand if she was dying!

I give women credit for knowing the difference between a sexual hug and a friendly hug. Gynecologists don't see a pelvic exam as a sexual experience; we understand that it can be extremely awkward and embarrassing for the patient. So there are times when we hold your hand or put our arms around you after the exam to let you know we care. That's not a sexual thing to do; it is certainly no more personal than putting our hands inside your vagina during the exam. Of course, if your doctor ever touches you in a way that makes you feel uncomfortable, tell him. But remember that comforting patients is a natural part of caring for them, at least among those doctors who haven't lost the human touch.

What rights do you have to your medical records?

How do your medical records play a part in the doctor-patient partnership? Most patients never consider requesting a copy of their records unless they are having problems obtaining medical insurance, are switching doctors, or are planning to sue their doctor. But if you and your gynecologist are truly to work together as a team, then your medical records are a tool to which both of you should have access.

What do medical records contain, and why would it serve you as a patient to have copies of them? These records, which are written by your doctor, usually include the medical history form you filled out at your first appointment; notes taken at each visit about your condition and any physical problems; your diagnosis and a list of medications or other treatments; copies of lab test results; any personal comments the doctor has recorded about you; information from any consulting physicians; and medical insurance information. If you are hospitalized, your medical chart for each hospitalization contains similar records. Since your rights to your doctor's records and hospital records are very similar, I will refer here—for the sake of simplicity—only to your doctor's records.

To be an informed patient and an active participant in your care, you must have copies of your records. You can refer to this information to help you remember and understand what the doctor tells you about your condition, diagnosis, and treatment. It can serve as an educational tool, helping your doctor to better inform you and helping you to ask better questions. As we saw in Chapter 2 (and will discuss further in Chapter 4), you can verify that your doctor received the results of your lab tests and not those of another person with a similar name, and that you understand the findings of the tests.

Most patients still don't know they have the right to see their medical records, and a surprising number of doctors believe that it is within their right to deny a patient access to her file. True, the originals of your records are the property of the individual physician. But in almost every case and almost every state, no law prohibits you from having copies of those records. If a doctor tells you it is illegal to have a copy of your records, he should be able to cite the legal statute involved. Your doctor may ask you to put your request for copies of your records in writing, but you don't need to justify the request. He will usually ask you to sign a release form. An ethical doctor will only charge you for the photocopying costs, without additional clerical fees.

Your first visit to a new physician is a good time to inform the doctor that you want copies of your records. You can do this by writing "Please send copies of all records to me" on the patient application form.

> Unless you've had a bad experience, you probably never think of asking to see your records. During my regular checkup, my gynecologist told me I had a pelvic mass, but he just told me to double up on my hormone pills and see him in another month. That didn't sound right to me, so a friend referred me to another doctor for a second opinion. He found several masses, and sent me straight away to get a sonogram. The second doctor put through an urgent request for my medical records, but got no response. In surgery the following morning, I was found to have a seeping ovarian cyst; if it had broken open, I could have died of peritonitis. It turned out that my original doctor had known for a year that I had ovarian cysts. While I was still in the hospital, he sent me a nasty letter calling me neurotic. But it took twenty-eight days for him to release my records to the second doctor—who was only one block away.
>
> —Megan, an administrative assistant

If you request a copy of your records and your doctor tells you the information won't mean anything to you, you might respond this way: "I know I'm not a doctor and I'm not questioning your expertise, but I don't know enough to ask the right questions of you. After I look over the information in the records, I'll be able to ask you the proper questions." Should your doctor still resist, you can respond "Dr. X, I'm paying you for this service." He may also say that he will only release the records to another doctor, but insist on your rights—and put them in writing. If you follow the proper procedures for obtaining copies of the records and still get no response, you can say "Dr. X, I'm sending you a letter that says I want copies of all my records because I'm dismissing myself from your care."

Getting a second opinion

Early in my career, I felt one of my patients needed surgery; her insurance company required a second opinion. I'd been her gynecologist for two years, and she was very apprehensive about going to someone else. However, I encouraged her to go. The physician, whom I had not met, called me to suggest that a particular new antibiotic might solve her problem instead of surgery. That antibiotic hadn't occurred to me, but I agreed with him. Well, the patient was furious that Dr. No. 2 had, in her opinion, underestimated the trust and loyalty she felt for me. I had to convince her to try his solution. The antibiotics did the trick and she avoided surgery, but to this day she dislikes that doctor. I, on the other hand, became good friends with him because I respected his judgment and appreciated his honesty and concern for my patient. We need many more doctors who will stand up and say to a colleague, "I believe you haven't thought of this."

While your doctor isn't obligated to suggest that you get another opinion, it is absolutely your right to get a second opinion, a third opinion, or as many medical opinions as you want. Insurance companies may require second opinions, and even if they don't require one for your particular treatment, they will usually cover the expenses if you request one.

How do you get a second opinion? Let's refer to your regular physician as Dr. No. 1 and the doctor you consult for a second opinion as Dr. No. 2. To get an honest second opinion, first be honest with Dr. No. 1. A good doctor will not only graciously and courteously encourage you to seek a second opinion but will also provide copies of your x-rays and other records to the second physician, cooperating fully with him.

In all your dealings with Dr. No. 2, keep in mind that you want him to be as objective as possible. For this reason, don't go to Dr. No. 1's partner for a second opinion. Don't reveal more than is necessary to Dr. No. 2. In fact, don't make him aware that you've come to him for a second opinion. Some doctors are reluctant to give second opinions; if they are friends or work at the same hospital with your doctor, they may feel this is harassing a colleague. And since you want Dr. No. 2 to be as unbiased as possible, you don't want him to know Dr. No. 1's diagnosis or recommended treatment. Don't tell him "My own doctor suggests I undergo this procedure." Simply tell him you want an examination and describe your symptoms.

What if Dr. No. 1 has already run a series of tests, and Dr. No. 2 tells you he needs to run the same tests in order to make a diagnosis? You may not be able to avoid showing Dr. No. 2 your test results, particularly if the tests are too costly or involve too many risks to repeat. In that case, remember that it's all right to share information between doctors. So if Dr. No. 1 has already done a blood count, you have the right to say to Dr. No. 2 "Don't retest me. I think I've had that. Would you please call the doctor I usually go to?" Doctors share information all the time, as we all know how expensive medical care is for the patient these days. On the other hand, if you are considering having a serious operation and the tests involved are not overly expensive or risky, it might be better to let Dr. No. 2 repeat them. After all, if you're talking about redoing a few x-rays, how do you know that the x-ray department Dr. No. 1 used is a good one, or that your x-rays were read correctly? If you've had a tissue biopsy, I would not recommend you repeat it, but you can have the slides reviewed by another pathologist; the same goes for Pap smear slides. But don't tell the pathologist your doctor's name; the pathologist might have some negative or positive opinion about your doctor that could weigh in his findings.

If you must let Dr. No. 2 know that you've come to him for a second opinion, a good physician will respect your desire for another opinion. However, it would be unproductive to say "I want a second opinion about whether or not I need a hysterectomy." Not only will you compromise Dr. No. 2's objectivity, but he is likely to ask who's going to operate on you; and if he has a strong opinion about that person, he will be even more biased.

Since both doctors have had the same information to go on, they should reach the same conclusions. Therefore, if Dr. No. 1 has told you that you need a hysterectomy, but Dr. No. 2 doesn't agree, you may need to seek a third opinion. It is your right to investigate all of your options, and it is your responsibility to gather information until you feel you are informed enough to make the choice that is right for you.

> I wasn't feeling well, and I just felt my gynecologist wasn't trying to help me. She didn't even return my phone calls. Even so, it took me forever to get up the nerve to go to another doctor for a second opinion. When I requested that a copy of my medical reports be sent to the other doctor, that would have been a perfect time for her to ask me why I felt I needed a second opinion. I had every intention of going back to her. I liked her, and she had good credentials. But she wouldn't talk to me after that. She was furious that I was consulting another doctor. I felt really awful and guilty for a while. The second doctor found out what the problem was, and put me in the hospital for surgery. My former doctor called my new doctor to ask

if she was going to get sued. She never apologized or visited me at the hospital to see how I was doing. That's all I would have wanted.

—Madeline, a computer technincian

How do you find a good gynecologist?

While I was putting together the material for this section, I thought it would be interesting to do an informal survey among my patients as well as some of the nurses I know. When I put this question to one patient, she said, "Do you want to know how I think women really look for gynecologists, or how they *should* look for them?" What was the difference? I asked. "How women really look for doctors is the way I looked for one before I became educated," she replied.

This sounded interesting, so I asked a number of these women to tell me what hadn't worked for them in the past. Referrals by word of mouth was the consensus. The one who best summed up their responses said, "A friend of mine asked me not long ago if I knew of a good gynecologist. If I had said, 'I got one out of the phone book,' she would have responded, 'I trust you because you're my friend, and that's the only recommendation I need.' Here someone will trust their health care to a doctor recommended by a friend, simply because of the strength and trust of the friendship."

On the issue of credentials, one patient aptly summed up the inability of most patients to evaulate the professional background of a gynecologist.

> I went to doctors based on whether they operated out of a facility with a good reputation, and by the credentials and medical reputation of the doctor. I found that didn't necessarily help me at all. After going to someone who was very highly recommended and well respected, my medical problem wasn't going away. Not only that,

but I felt that I was being treated condescendingly, that I was being told that I had no problem when I knew I did. You can have a doctor who has all the credentials in the world, and they don't mean anything if he doesn't listen, if he can't treat the person as well as the symptoms. There's got to be a balance."

—Morgan, a sales clerk

Before you begin to look for a gynecologist, you have a number of decisions to make. One of the most basic is the setting in which you will receive gynecological care. Do you want a doctor in private practice? If so, would a solo practitioner meet your needs, or would you prefer a group practice?

If you are a member of a Health Maintenance Organization (HMO) or a Preferred Provider Organization (PPO), will you be satisfied to have a family doctor or internist provide your routine gynecological care, or can you choose to have both a family doctor and a gynecologist? Do you belong to the type of HMO called an Individual Practice Association (IPA), which would allow you to have a doctor who works out of a private office rather than a centralized location?

Clinics are another alternative for many women. Since the 1960s, a small number of "womancare" centers have been founded to give women control over their health care. Women's health care clinics are another alternative, but don't assume that they are independent or offer better care than other settings; many serve as profit centers for hospitals. Hospital clinics are a boon to women who cannot afford a private physician, but they are also classrooms for young doctors.

You owe it to yourself to do the same homework on a group health organization or clinic as you would on an individual gynecologist. Above all, in every setting where gynecological care is offered, my advice to patients is the same: ask questions, and then ask more questions, until you are satisfied that your doctor has informed you fully about your diagnosis and the alternatives for treatment.

I wish I could tell you some shortcuts to choosing a gynecologist, but there are none. There is no place you can call
to find the names of good gynecologists or those you
should avoid. Besides, the right gynecologist for you is the
one who meets your own special needs, so you alone are
equipped to make the choice. I can, however, make some
suggestions to guide you through the selection process.

There are at least four stages to the process of selecting a
gynecologist. First, you need to set some parameters. What
factors or characteristics are most important to you? Second,
draw up a list of suitable candidates. Third, gain whatever
information you can about them before you meet them.
Finally, visit their offices and interview them personally.

While you alone must set priorities among the many factors you could consider, here are some questions to ask
yourself:

- Would I prefer a solo practitioner or a doctor in a
  group practice?
- Do I want a gynecologist who is also a practicing
  obstetrician?
- Do I want a gynecologist who will also provide primary care, or would I rather go to a family physician,
  general practitioner, or internist for my general health
  needs?
- Do I have a particular medical problem, such as infertility or cancer, that might call for my having a specialist
  as my regular gynecologist?
- Does it matter to me whether my gynecologist is male
  or female?
- Is it important to me that my doctor be board-certified
  in gynecology?
- Do I want my gynecologist to have privileges at a particular hospital?
- How much importance do I place on a doctor's bedside manner and on her technical ability?

When you are making up your list of candidates, it's perfectly acceptable to start by getting referrals from your
friends, co-workers, or relatives. Draw them out on why
they chose that particular doctor and what they like and
dislike about him or her. If possible, seek out referrals from
other doctors whom you respect. Physician-referral services
can provide names of gynecologists who are accepting new
patients, but bear in mind that these doctors have paid to
be included.

> As a nurse, it really upsets me that women would
> use the Yellow Pages to choose a gynecologist. If I was
> new to an area and didn't know anyone who could
> refer me to a doctor, I'd find a hospital with a good
> reputation, and call the gynecological floor at that
> hospital. I'd ask to talk to a staff or floor nurse, and I'd
> call at different times so I would reach nurses on the
> day shift as well as the night shift. If I couldn't get
> enough nurses to talk to me on the phone, I'd go in
> person. Nurses work with doctors every day; they
> know whose patients do well in the hospital and are
> better informed, and they see which doctors spend
> time with their patients. A nurse isn't supposed to rec-
> ommend or refer doctors, but you can ask who is her
> own gynecologist. If you ask enough nurses, pretty
> soon you'll hear the same doctors' names coming up.
> —Penny, a nurse at a major metropolitan
>   hospital

You can do some homework before you meet any of
your candidates. To find out which gynecologists in your
area are board-certified or have a particular specialty, check
your library for the *Directory of Medical Specialists,* published by the American Board of Medical Specialties
(ABMS). This reference will also tell you where a doctor did
his residency training and how long he has been practicing.

You can find out if a candidate on your list is licensed to practice medicine in your state by calling your state's medical licensing board. This board can also tell you whether they have taken disciplinary action against a particular doctor, but they usually won't reveal whether his license has been revoked in another state, or whether he has had malpractice charges filed against him.

When you call each prospective doctor's office, the manner in which his staff handles your call will give you a clue as to his own interaction with patients. Get answers to the following questions:

- Is this doctor accepting new patients?
- What are his office hours?
- Does he accept Medicare assignment?
- Can he provide a list of his basic fees?
- At which hospitals does he work?
- Does he take phone calls from patients personally?
- To whom does he refer his patients when he is on vacation or otherwise unavailable?
- Does he accept my medical insurance?
- How much time does he allocate for yearly examinations? For first visits?
- Does he take get-acquainted appointments? If so, how much time will he spend with me and what will he charge?

To find a gynecologist who will work with you as a partner, the get-acquainted visit is the most crucial step you can take.

When I was looking for a gynecologist, I made appointments for consults. One doctor wouldn't agree to see me unless I was definitely going to become a patient. I crossed him off the list. The next candidate wouldn't let my husband come into the office with me. He too got dropped from my list. The third gynecologist I went to see saw me on his lunch hour. We spent that whole hour talking in his office. Out of that lunch hour, he gained a new patient, and I gained a wonderful doctor.

—Lisa, a hospital nurse

While you size up a gynecologist during your initial interview, you can be looking for answers to the following questions:

- What kind of reception did I get from his office staff?
- Was he on time for his appointment with me?
- Does he seem willing to spend time with me?
- Does he look me straight in the eye and speak frankly to me?
- Is he a good listener? How often does he interrupt me?
- Does he seem genuinely interested in me as a person?
- Does he provide informative answers to my questions, or do his answers seem vague, rehearsed, or overly general?
- Do I feel a rapport with him?
- Do I feel I could discuss the intimate details of my sexual and emotional life with him?

Medical qualifications aside, you have to decide whether you can communicate with the person you choose as your gynecologist. Once you choose a person you think will work with you, keep going until you feel comfortable asking them your questions. If it doesn't feel good, be honest with yourself and know that you have to go somewhere else. If it takes going to five or six different doctors until you find the right match, it will be worth it.

How to switch doctors

Women often feel guilty for switching doctors. Not only do they feel a strong sense of loyalty, but they are apt to take responsibility for their doctor's reaction: "My doctor will feel bad if I leave." Don't focus on your doctor's feelings. You're the consumer; you have a right to try a new "brand."

Once you've decided to switch doctors, you have the right to get copies of your medical records, even if you have an outstanding balance. You can handle this in one of two ways. Call the doctor's office in advance to say that you will be coming by to pick up copies of your records, and that you will sign a medical release to that effect; send a brief letter (or have your new physician do this for you, with your signature) requesting that a copy of all your records be sent either to you or to the new physician. (You have a right to speedy delivery of those records.)

> Even though the need was clear to me, it took me forever to switch doctors. My own fear was holding me back, because most of us are aware that doctors have egos. What went through my mind was, If I threaten his ego, what if he retaliates? What will he think of me? But then I told myself: What does it matter to me if this doctor thinks I'm neurotic or bitchy? Having a doctor I can trust could, some day, be a matter of life or death.
>
> —Jean, an insurance agent

To speak frankly, I think patients are often a little too quick to see their doctors as close friends. Jean is correct about the egos of doctors. We tend to feel that our patients belong to us. When a patient wants to switch, it bothers even the best of us. Good physicians try to rise above that, learn from the experience, and become better doctors. When you demand the best from your doctor and switch if necessary to receive proper care, you will make things that much better for other women.

CHAPTER 4

The Gynecological Exam and the Pap Smear: What They Reveal

Questions you may never have asked—but should have

Let's face it, you don't look forward to having a gynecological exam any more than you look forward to filing your tax return. But now that we've established that you and your gynecologist must work together as partners and that it's your responsiblity to participate in your own health care, you can feel much more in control of the situation. How do you put this health-promoting partnership into practice? The "gyn" exam, as we'll call it, is where it all happens. In addition to its being the doctor's annual assessment of your body to detect changes since your last visit or abnormalities that could become serious if left untreated, it's also your opportunity to educate and inform yourself. Through the exchange of questions and answers between you and your doctor, you are able—as partners—to make choices on behalf of your reproductive health and emotional well-being.

For a frank discussion covering a young woman's first gynecological examination, see "A Word to Young Women" in the Appendix.

Who needs to have routine gyn exams and how often? The American College of Obstetrics and Gynecology, the American Cancer Society, and the National Cancer Institute are in agreement that all women who are, have been, or may soon be sexually active, or who are planning to become pregnant, as well as all women who have reached age eighteen, should have an annual pelvic examination and Pap test. A young woman should also come in for her first exam if she has a vaginal discharge or is experiencing menstrual problems such as pain or abnormal bleeding.

> A lot of women still don't think of this whole arena as a matter of life or death. I work with a very intelligent, twenty-eight-year-old college graduate. One day I mentioned that I had to leave early for my annual gynecology checkup, and she said, "I've just never done that yet." Because she is my friend, I answered, "Haven't you ever had sex?" And she said, "Of course." "Well, you're about twelve years too late!" I told her. So she took the money she was saving to buy a VCR and went to a doctor instead. I think a lot of people are like my friend. They'll go to the dentist because they know their teeth hurt, but they could have a serious problem like cancer and never know it.
>
> —Ellen, a research scientist

If you or your partner have had any sexually transmitted diseases (STDs), or if you are unsure of your partner's sexual history, I strongly urge you to get at least a yearly pelvic exam and Pap smear. The cost can't begin to compare with the risk of contracting one of the many STDs, which are so widespread and potentially deadly if left undetected.

Don't wait for your annual exam. Instead, see your gynecologist at once if you experience severe abdominal pain, vaginal hemorrhaging, or pain in conjunction with a missed or late period. You should see your doctor as soon as possible if you develop:

- Lower abdominal pain
- Severe menstrual cramps
- Bleeding and/or pain during intercourse
- Excessive menstrual bleeding or bleeding between periods
- Irregular or missed periods
- Breast lumps
- Vaginal itching or burning, and/or changes in a vaginal discharge
- Sores in your genital or anal region

Everything that follows about the gyn exam and Pap smear applies no matter whether you go to a private physician, see a gynecologist through an HMO (Health Maintenance Organization) or PPO (Preferred Provider Organization), or go to any kind of women's health clinic. Certain clinics are run by professional nurse practitioners, who have the expertise and the legal right to examine patients and, in some states, to write prescriptions. If a nurse practitioner or another type of health care provider examines you, this person is acting as an agent of a physician, and you have the same rights and responsibilities as those covered in this and the previous chapter.

Preparation for your appointment

When you are having a gyn exam, your responsibility to ask questions begins when you first call a gynecologist's office to make the appointment. Even if you have already made a get-acquainted visit to this doctor's office (see Chapter 3), you are still in the process of evaluating whether he or she is the right doctor for you. This is your opportunity to ask any questions that you didn't raise during your get-acquainted interview, and there are things you need to know before you come in for your examination. In most cases, the receptionist or nurse should be able to answer the following questions:

What is the approximate cost of an annual exam and Pap test?

Depending on the outcome of your examination, your doctor may need to do extra cultures or procedures that will add to the charges, but his office should be able to quote a basic fee. Similarly, you've probably left a hair salon with $30 worth of products that you hadn't planned on buying, but at least you found out in advance how much your haircut or perm was going to cost.

Is payment expected at the time of the visit? Do you take my health plan? Do you take care of insurance forms and the filing of claims?

If you go to a physician whose office won't answer questions on charges and insurance coverage, you could end up with a bill that you cannot afford to pay. (Besides, why would you buy a product if you didn't know how much it cost?)

When going to a clinic: Who is your medical director and how often does he see the patients' charts? Will I be examined by a physician, a physician-in-training, or a nurse practitioner?

If the medical director doesn't review charts frequently or only reviews charts of those patients whose lab tests were flagged as abnormal, find another clinic. Labs aren't infallible, and you need to know that a physician is keeping a sharp eye on your case.

Where do you send your Pap smears?

Does the doctor have any financial interest in the laboratory? See the discussion titled "The pap test" later in this chapter.

Does this gynecologist make it a practice to consult with patients before they get undressed for the exam?

If not, have the receptionist ask the doctor whether he will agree to make this a standard procedure in your case. If he will, thank him when you meet with him, and tell him why you feel this will help you communicate with him better. By speaking up, you will educate him and thus benefit other women. If he won't agree to meet with you with your clothes on before and after the exam, politely let him know that this is the reason you will not be seeing him as a patient. Again, whether you tell him over the phone, or write him a letter, you will be doing your part as a consumer to educate this doctor.

How much time will the appointment take?

Let the person who sets up appointments know your purpose for the visit. State any health problems you want to discuss beforehand so your doctor can allot adequate time; you won't receive the attention you deserve if you bring up issues as an afterthought.

If this will be the first time you have ever had a gynecological exam or your first exam from a new gynecologist, ask that you be scheduled for a longer appointment than usual. As a guideline, a new-patient appointment should take at least an hour. A routine exam, if you have seen this doctor previously, will run about thirty to forty-five minutes. Unless you have a medical problem, you will see your physician only once a year. Be sure you and your doctor allocate enough time so that you don't feel rushed.

Can my partner or a friend be present during the appointment? If I desire, can they be present during the examination?

Your doctor should be flexible enough to accommodate your wishes. If you want someone along for moral support, that's your right. Your gynecologist should be especially pleased if your spouse or partner is willing to come in and ask any questions he has about sexually transmitted diseases, sexuality, reproduction, or even basic anatomy. However, doctors know that sometimes husbands or partners want to be present during the gyn exam out of possessiveness or to prevent any talk of physical or sexual abuse. Your doctor's first concern is that you are able to talk freely, and he is duty-bound to respect your privacy and maintain confidentiality. Let him know ahead of time that your partner will accompany you, and under what circumstances you want your partner present—or absent—when you are talking to your doctor.

Is a chaperone usually in the room during the physical examination?

In my opinion, a chaperone should be present regardless of the sex of the doctor. There are several advantages to having someone serve as a chaperone. That person can assist the physician, and if the gynecologist is male, having another woman in the room may help the patient feel less uncomfortable. The presence of a chaperone also eliminates any potential for inappropriate behavior on the part of either the doctor or the patient. Most doctors and patients would never engage in unsuitable conduct, but a chaperone keeps everybody honest. By serving as a third pair of ears, the chaperone can help correct any miscommunication between doctor and patient and can later answer a patient's questions, should the doctor be unavailable.

At what point in my cycle should I schedule an appointment?

If at all possible, schedule your exam for a time when you are not having your menstrual period. (Come prepared to tell your doctor the date your last period began.) A Pap smear is best taken two weeks before your period. But if you are experiencing excessive menstrual bleeding, let your doctor know, as he may want to examine you during your period. Your doctor won't think twice about checking you during your flow, so you need not feel embarrassed.

Do I need to do anything to prepare for the physical part of the examination?

It is important that you do not douche or use any vaginal medicine twenty-four hours before the exam, as this could affect the results of your Pap smear. If you have any questions about this, call before the day of your appointment.

There is one final step to take before you come in for your appointment. To be sure that you don't forget anything you want to cover during your exam, make out a list ahead of time. This list could include symptoms or health problems you are experiencing. Add other concerns you want the doctor to check you for, including the possibility that you may have acquired an STD. Also, write down topics and questions you want to discuss so you become a better-informed patient. If you want to get the most out of the time your doctor will spend in educating you, read up on topics that may relate to your care. The newsstands are full of magazines with articles about women's health care, STDs, sexuality, and so on.

Preliminaries at your doctor's office

If this is your first visit, you will probably have to fill out some paperwork, such as a medical history, as well as supply information on your insurance carrier. All information you supply to your doctor's office is confidential. If you have any special requests, be sure to attach them to this paperwork. As we've discussed, one request you should certainly put in writing is that you want all Pap test lab reports to be sent to you. "Do not call me at work" and, in the case of a younger patient, "do not send reports to my parents' home" are examples of requests you might make.

While individual practices vary, you will probably undergo a few basic procedures before you meet with your doctor. A staff member will check your weight and blood pressure; take a blood sample for a blood count and possibly a cholesterol check; and ask you to provide a urine sample (typically analyzed for signs of diabetes or problems involving the bladder or kidneys).

Talking with your gynecologist before the physical exam

At this point, if you have done your homework on this gynecologist, he should—without prompting—usher you into a private office. He will have a number of questions to ask you, and you should have questions of your own. Your doctor's goal for this discussion is not only to learn about your health but to educate you. Unless he's a mind-reader, however, he'll have to rely on you to tell him what your questions and concerns are. Like you, doctors can be shy. Don't waste the one hour per year you spend face-to-face with your gynecologist: be open, honest, and thorough.

Now is the time for you to elaborate on the medical history form you completed earlier. Remember that everything you tell your doctor is strictly confidential and will be used solely to determine the best medical care for you. He will ask about your family medical history and your own medical, gynecological, and surgical history. It is important to tell him about any medications you are taking and about any to which you are allergic. Understand that he will need to ask whether you smoke or use drugs or alcohol.

This is also the time when your gynecologist should ask about your sexual history and sexual behavior. Hide nothing in your history, including pregnancies, abortions, or STDs you have had. Tell him in detail about your birth control methods. He'll also ask how many partners you have had and about the specific sexual practices in which you have engaged. His purpose in doing so is not to pry into your personal life or to embarrass you, but rather to find out what risks, if any, you have been exposed to, and to gain the best possible understanding of your medical needs.

> Seldom do women give much thought to what questions to ask their gynecologist. Some of my patients who come in for an exam apologize for having a list of questions. I tell them right off, "Don't apologize, that's

wonderful! If you have in mind what you want to get out of your session, and what questions you have, we're ten steps ahead of the game."

—Anne, a gynecologist in the Seattle area

Many of the questions you should raise during your conversation prior to the pelvic exam have to do with the Pap smear. A list of these important questions will accompany our discussion about the Pap test later in this chapter.

Here are some additional questions to ask your gynecologist during your initial talk:

- What procedures will the exam include, and what will you be looking for?
- Do you routinely screen for any sexually transmitted diseases? If so, which STDs do you screen for, and how much will each test cost?

As we'll discuss in detail later, certain STDs are both rampant and dangerous but unfortunately have few or no symptoms. Even so, the majority of gynecologists don't routinely test for most STDs. The problem is compounded by patients' assumptions that these tests are included in a routine exam.

Sometimes it's hard for a doctor to suggest STD testing because he knows it's going to cost extra. Don't let anyone tell you that because you have no symptoms, it's not worthwhile to be tested. The cost of STD testing is cheaper by far than what the complications of an STD will cost.

It is up to you, the patient, to educate yourself about STDs and to demand that you be tested for them. A good doctor will ask you why you want to be tested. This pre-exam dialogue with your doctor is the best time for you to discuss any possibility that you may have contracted an STD and what tests you may need.

This talk is also an opportunity for your doctor to get to know you as a person. Good doctors don't just treat bodies, they treat people. Not all doctors are comfortable with or skilled at interpersonal communication, so it is your responsibility to tell your doctor about any aspect of your life that may be having an effect on your health. If your doctor identifies a problem that he isn't trained to deal with, he should be able to give you an appropriate referral.

> I saw a patient who just didn't look good. She complained of lumps in her groin, adding that her cramps had been really bad the past few months, although they'd been fine before that. I said, "Gee, that's kind of strange. Is something going on? Something different?" She started to cry but didn't want to talk about it. So I asked, "Is the problem at work or at home?" We gradually got to what was going on, a family problem, and I referred her to a therapist. She said she couldn't afford one, but I said, "You can't afford not to see somebody. You're falling apart, you have some decisions to make, and trying to handle this alone isn't working." She eventually agreed to put her "cigarette" money toward getting some help.
>
> —Gwen, a gynecologist in private practice

When your doctor has answered all your questions to your satisfaction, it is time for the next stage in your visit, the gynecological examination. It is natural for many women to feel a little nervous about this exam. However, if your questions have all been answered and you still have any strong fears about the exam itself, now is the time to share them with your doctor. Ask him to take whatever steps he can to minimize the discomfort.

> When I was in my twenties, I used to go to a clinic to save money. They dispensed birth control and required an annual physical, including blood-work and a Pap smear. At the time I didn't think I needed all that; I just wanted my pills. Then I turned up with an abnor-

mal Pap test and went through treatment for an STD. Today I'd say that if you're going to have an annual exam, even if you don't go to a private gynecologist, go someplace where they do an all-over, thorough exam. I would never be satisfied with a place that essentially takes your blood and then dispenses birth control. I'd make sure they did everything a regular gynecologist did, and that there was a doctor supervising the patient care in the clinic.

Kathy, a flight attendant

The basic gynecological examination

After you have undressed in private and put on an examination gown or wrap, your gynecologist and the chaperone will enter the examining room. Your doctor will probably begin by checking your general health. She may examine your neck, ears, nose, and throat; check your heart and lungs with a stethoscope; examine your thyroid gland (located at the base of your neck); and check the lymph nodes in your neck, armpits, and groin. She will do a breast examination and may choose to order a mammogram (x-ray examination of the breasts). If you don't know how to examine your own breasts, ask her to demonstrate. This is an important skill to learn, as most tumors are detected by monthly self-examination. Palpating (feeling and gently pressing) your abdomen, she will check your liver, spleen, and other areas for abnormal growths or tenderness.

The genital and pelvic examination

Now your gynecologist will do a number of procedures to check the condition of your external and internal female organs. For this she will ask you to scoot down to the end of the examining table so that you are lying on your back in a squatting position, and to place your feet in stirrups at either side of the table. As vulnerable as this position makes you feel, it gives your doctor the clearest view to inspect your genital region and allows the room she will need to perform the internal exam. The doctor may put a drape over your legs, but if you would rather be uncovered so that you can see her face and what is taking place, she should honor your preference. Many patients find it reassuring if their gynecologist describes what she is doing and finding every step of the way. You can also ask her to give you a hand mirror or position a mirror so that you can see what's happening; ask her to point out anything you have questions about.

Wearing surgical gloves, the doctor will start by inspecting your external genitals, including the *mons pubis* (the mound covered by pubic hair), the *labia majora* and *labia minora* (outer and inner vaginal lips), the *clitoris* (sensitive knob at the top of the vaginal lips), the *Bartholin glands* (lubricating glands on each side of the vagina), the *urethra* (urinary opening), and the vaginal opening. She will be looking for irritation, changes in skin color or moles, genital warts, herpes and other sores, or any signs of a genital infection or other abnormal condition.

Next, the doctor will probably tell you to relax. This is a nonsensical statement, since we know it's not going to help you relax and will probably have the opposite effect. But if you take long, slow breaths, hopefully your pelvic muscles will relax and allow her to gently insert a *speculum* into your vagina. This is a metal or plastic device resembling a duckbill; once inserted, the sides are locked open about an inch apart. The speculum enables the doctor to view your cervix (the neck of the uterus, which extends into the vagina) and to insert and withdraw instruments without touching the sides of your vagina.

Unless you have a vaginal or other internal infection, or sores in your vagina, the insertion of the speculum and the internal exam should not be painful, although it is normally a little uncomfortable. Speculums come in several different sizes. Some procedures (such as biopsies) call for a larger speculum. If your last exam was uncomfortable, ask your doctor if it is possible to use a smaller speculum; your vagina may be smaller than your outward size indicates. Considerate gynecologists will warm the speculum before insertion.

The first procedure is usually a sampling of the cervix called a Pap smear, which we will discuss shortly.

If you want your gynecologist to do any tests for STDs such as chlamydia or gonorrhea, this is the time, while the speculum is in place. If for some reason you haven't discussed STD testing up to this point, it is still a simple matter for your doctor to perform. As with the Pap smear, these tests are relatively quick and painless.

As your doctor withdraws the speculum, she may rotate it slightly so that she can make a visual examination of the vagina for any infection or abnormalities. She will also make sure that the glands supplying moisture to the vagina are free of disease.

In the second part of the pelvic exam, your gynecologist will palpate your internal genital organs, looking for any abnormalities. To do this, she will insert one or two gloved and lubricated fingers into your vagina while pressing with her other hand on your lower abdomen. She will check your ovaries (one on each side), fallopian tubes, and uterus for any tender or enlarged areas, and for any growths. It is normal during this part of the exam for you to be slightly uncomfortable, as your doctor must press deeply on your abdomen. You may also feel a pinching pain in one ovary if you are mid-cycle and ovulating. However, should the exam feel unduly uncomfortable, let your doctor know. And if you have not previously told your doctor that you experience pain during intercourse or at other times, it is very important to inform her now, as this may suggest the need to check you for diseases such as endometriosis.

Keeping one finger in your vagina, your gynecologist will probably now insert another finger into your rectum and ask you to bear down. In this way she can properly evaluate the back side of the uterus and the space between your vagina and rectum, which is hard to check otherwise; she can also better examine your ovaries. Because this procedure can help her to detect rectal growths, cancer, and other diseases, its importance outweighs the temporary discomfort and embarrassment you may feel.

The follow-up talk

Now the physical examination is completed; but your appointment isn't over. It's time to discuss the preliminary findings and how your test results will be handled. Let your doctor know that you want this talk to take place after you are dressed, and in her office.

Patients often come up with more questions during this second talk, after they've had a chance to sift through what was discussed earlier. Just as before the exam, your doctor should answer all your questions and concerns or should set up another appointment for this purpose.

Be sure to reiterate that you want the actual lab report on your Pap smear (as well as any other STD tests) mailed to you. We'll talk about why this is so important shortly. Also, find out how long this will take, so you won't be waiting apprehensively if you don't get the results within a day or two.

Abnormal findings

Should your examination uncover a problem, know that gynecology is just about the only specialty in which we can say that if there *is* bad news, we can probably fix it. If you have regular checkups, we can diagnose almost all problems at a stage when they can be treated.

As always, the quality of the care you receive rests on the questions you ask. If your doctor suspects or has diagnosed a problem, you'll need to ask a lot of questions. You may want to come back another time, accompanied by someone who can listen objectively and raise questions that may not occur to you. Here are some questions to include:

- Can I look forward to a complete recovery? How long will recovery take? How is this problem going to affect my life six months from now? A year from now? Ten years from now?
- Why are you recommending this treatment (drug, operation, etc.)? If patients understand why their doctor wants them to take some action, they are much more likely to comply.
- What could happen to me if I don't do anything about this? That's an important question. There may be no harm in tolerating your symptoms and waiting to see what happens. On the other hand, if you were to do nothing, you might end up infertile or with invasive cervical cancer.
- Do you have any written information about this problem I can take with me?

When your doctor recommends medication, here are some questions to ask her:

- What problem am I being given this drug for, and how is it supposed to work in my body?
- What are the possible risks and side effects of this drug?
- How should this drug be taken? Can it be taken in such a way as to minimize side effects?
- How will this drug interact with any other medications I am taking, either prescription drugs or over-the-counter remedies? Are there any other harmful interactions, such as with alcohol or any method of birth control, that I should know about? For example, some antibiotics may lower the effectiveness of birth control pills.
- Are there safer alternatives, either other drugs or a non-drug treatment, that would work just as well?

See also Chapter 16 if your doctor suggests surgery for further diagnosis or treatment.

After this talk is concluded, you will proceed to the receptionist, where you will be expected to make payment or to conclude any other payment arrangements that have been made. Check the bill for accuracy and make sure that you get a receipt. You may also want to double-check on procedures for handling insurance or other paperwork.

The Pap test

The Pap test is probably the most important part of your gynecological exam. "Pap" is short for Dr. George Papanicolaou, the physician who developed this test in the 1940s. He found that if a sample of cells from the cervix is analyzed under a microscope, a trained eye can detect the presence of cells that, if left undisturbed, might become cancerous. As we go along, keep in mind that a Pap smear does not provide a diagnosis; it does, however, give your doctor an idea that abnormalities are present and further testing is needed.

If the following discussion reminds you of a biology textbook, I hope you will stay with me. We need to cover some terms pertaining to the anatomy of your cervix, so that later on you will be able to make sense out of your own Pap test lab report. Remember Diane, who was never told that her Pap smears showed abnormalities, and who ultimately died of cervical cancer (see Introduction)? Do you recall Lesley, whose doctor wrote at the top of her Pap test report not to tell her that she had precancerous cells caused by exposure to a sexually transmitted disease (see Chapter 2)? Armed with the information that follows, you will be able to understand enough of your Pap test report to ask the questions that could save you from similar ordeals.

The *cervix* is the visible end of your uterus, or womb. It looks like a small doughnut; the hole in the middle is the opening to the *cervical canal,* which leads into the uterus. The cervix is covered with scalelike *squamous* cells; the cervical canal is lined with tall *columnar (glandular, endocervical)* cells. The zone where these two kinds of cells meet is called the *transformation zone (T-zone),* which is where abnormal cells are most likely to develop. Because the T-zone is more exposed on the cervix of women under thirty, they are especially susceptible to cervical infection.

Once again, the Pap test should be done about two weeks prior to your period, and you should not douche or insert any vaginal medicine for at least twenty-four hours prior to the test. To obtain a Pap smear, your gynecologist will take at least two cervical cell samples while you are lying on your back and the speculum is in place. Both samples are taken quickly and with only minor discomfort; you may notice a little spotting afterward.

Your doctor will gently scrape the outside of the cervix, called the *ectocervix,* with a tiny wooden or plastic spatula. He will also use a *cyto brush,* (also called an *endocervical brush* to scrape some cells from the inner canal of the cervix, called the *endocervical canal.* If your doctor does not use a cyto brush, she may miss precancerous cells or even cancers that are deep in the endocervical canal. You should feel a bit of scratching with both these tests. You *want* to feel that little scratch because it tells you the doctor is getting the best sample she can. A Pap smear done without a cyto brush should be considered a worthless Pap smear.

Your doctor will smear both samples onto a glass slide and spray the slide with a fixing solution to preserve them. Then they are sent to a laboratory, where technicians "read" them for evidence of early cancerous activity. Pap smears that are characterized as abnormal are then read by a pathologist, a physician who specializes in examining tissue for abnormalities.

Your best safeguards to ensure that your Pap smear is handled correctly are: first, that your gynecologist uses the proper sampling methods; and second, that she uses a competent lab. You can inquire about your doctor's sampling method, but how can you determine whether or not she uses a good lab? You would think that data would be available on a lab's accuracy rate—especially its false-negative rate—or on the number of Pap smears that each technician reads in a day. Realistically, even your gynecologist may not be able to come by this information. Until some qualified and impartial outside authority evaluates various labs and makes its findings available to the public, a layperson probably won't be able to answer this question fully.

However, as a patient, you can put into action your own form of quality control. It is crucial that you take the following steps:

1. Find out whether your gynecologist has a financial interest in the lab she uses.

This is something you should check out before you decide on a gynecologist. It may not be easy to ask this question, but wouldn't you want to know if there was a potential conflict of interest? This is just as legitimate and reasonable a question as asking whether your auto mechanic has a financial interest in the body shop he recommended to you. Your doctor should have no such tie to the lab she uses. That way, she has more incentive to choose a lab based on its competence.

2. Obtain your own copy of the Pap test lab report whether your Pap was normal or abnormal. This is not an option, but a responsibility, of every gynecological patient.

Why do you, a layperson, need a copy of the technical report from the lab? There are several reasons, and all are critical.

Let me start by asking, have you ever received Pap test results via a postcard in the mail? Postcard notification is misleading and risky. How do you know that the clerk who sent out the card didn't misfile your report or switch it with another patient's file whose name is similar to yours? I can think of one particular patient whom I'll call Ann Smith, who was referred to me with invasive cervical cancer. Ann's doctor had been sending her those little cards saying her Pap was normal. By coincidence her annual exam fell at the same time as that of another patient whose name was *Anne* Smith. She had been getting postcards that said her Pap was abnormal. You guessed it. Anne—the patient with the similar name—ended up having a biopsy she didn't need (because she actually had no abnormalities), and Ann found out she had cancer (which might have been prevented if it had been caught earlier).

If the sole issue here were how you should be notified whether your Pap smear is normal or abnormal, I would simply make the point that you have the right to notification over the phone and by your doctor. I don't want to belittle this right. What happened with Ann Smith is not an isolated incident; mistakes like that can happen in the best of practices when correspondence with patients (whether by postcard or form letter) is left to nonmedical staff. Because a gynecologist is more familiar with her patients than any clerk could be, she is far less likely to confuse one patient's name with another.

It is also your right, since confidentiality is part of the service you pay a gynecologist for, to get a call from your doctor, rather than a postcard that lets your mail carrier know the results of your Pap test. Once I received a postcard telling me when my back surgery was scheduled, and I remember thinking that it was none of the mail carrier's business to know that I was going to have an operation. Medical information should be confidential, and it is a breach of that confidentiality—let alone impolite—to treat it otherwise.

Before I leave the topic of notification, I want to make you aware of one of your most important rights. If your Pap smear is abnormal, your doctor—not a nurse or other staff person—has an obligation to call you. She alone has the expertise to answer all the questions you will undoubtedly have and to discuss what further tests might be needed. An abnormal Pap is upsetting news, but don't be intimidated; insist on speaking directly to your doctor. If a gynecologist isn't willing to spend a little time to tell you that your Pap smear was abnormal, how do you know she is going to take the time to give you proper care?

Assuming that your gynecologist always notifies you properly whether your Pap test was normal or abnormal, why do I insist that you obtain your own copy of the actual lab results? Certainly, you are the best person to double-check the patient name and social security number on the report to verify that it is indeed your Pap test report. To safe-guard your own health, you cannot place this responsibility solely in the hands of your doctor's office.

Most abnormal Pap smears are caused by sexually trans-mitted diseases. That is a fact no health practitioner can dis-pute, although not all gynecologists will say this so bluntly to patients. As I hope Chapter 2 clearly illustrates, many gyne-cologists fail to inform women that their medical problems are caused by STDs. In the case of abnormal Pap tests, countless women have been told to "wait and see" while their doctors kept an eye on their dysplasia (abnormal development or growth of cells, generally considered precancerous). Yet many of these women are never told that dysplasia is a sexually transmitted condition, which, if left untreated, can develop into cervical cancer. Without this information, women aren't in a position to know what questions to ask their doctors, and they don't know that their partners could keep reinfecting them unless they, too, are tested and treated.

Your doctor might withhold this kind of information from you out of the best of intentions, but that is not the point. For you to be a partner in your health care, you must have access to the same information about you that your doctor has, including the information in your lab reports and other medical records. When you can read your own Pap test lab report, you will know if the findings suggest that you should be tested for an STD; most of all, you will know what specific questions to ask your gynecologist.

Cassie is not a patient of mine, but she is a close friend. She and her new husband planned to have children eventually. Recently, after she visited her long-time gynecologist for a routine Pap smear, he told her that she needed a biopsy. "It's nothing you need to worry about," he insisted. "But what's the problem?" she asked. "Your Pap smear was abnormal for the second time in two years," he told her. "I'm really not concerned but we should check it out."

"The second time? Why wasn't I told about the first time? What exactly do you mean by abnormal?"

"Believe me. It's nothing serious."

Cassie made the appointment for the biopsy but left her doctor's office feeling confused and more than a little anxious. She called me, as a friend, to ask what I thought about all this. Not having seen any of her previous test results, I suggested that she get copies of all her lab reports, including the upcoming biopsy, so we could go over them together. I also suggested she ask her doctor whether he thought there was any chance her problem could be a sexually transmitted disease, in which case Cassie's husband should be examined as well.

When Cassie came in with her records, she had quite a story to tell. "I called my doctor's office and told the nurse I wanted copies of my lab reports. I also said that when I came in for the biopsy, I would need a few minutes to consult with the doctor before be began. On that day, however, he refused to see me until I was undressed. When he came

in, I asked whether my problem could be sexually transmitted. He just laughed and said that reading women's magazines didn't make me a doctor. I should have gotten dressed
and walked right out, but I went through with the biopsy.

"The next day, I returned to his office to get the results of
the biopsy and to retrieve my other records. At first this doctor—whom I had admired and trusted for so long—simply
refused to comply with my request. When I insisted, he closed
his office door and dropped to his knees. 'This is a molehill,'
he dramatized. Then he jumped to his feet and said, 'This is
a mountain.' Back down on his knees again, he said, 'Don't
turn your molehill into a mountain. You are fine.'

"His attempt to make a fool of me took me by surprise. I
probably wouldn't have thought to ask for my records on my
own accord, but it didn't seem like too much to ask. I just
wanted to know what was wrong with me. Right then I
decided that if my own doctor wouldn't explain this to me, I'd
go elsewhere. I demanded my records. He eventually turned
them over, but before he did, he made it clear I was no longer
welcome in his office. I had been labeled a 'difficult' patient."

After reviewing Cassie's records, I agreed with her former
doctor on one point. Her problem was not serious or life-
threatening, just a small infection. However, it could have
been sexually transmitted, so I suggested that her husband
be examined. If the problem was an STD and we only
treated Cassie, the infection would most likely recur and the
next time it could be more serious.

There was nothing embarrassing or uncomfortable about
our conversation. Cassie knew I wasn't suggesting that
either she or her husband were promiscuous. If a person
has had sex even once in her life without (and sometimes
even with) the use of a condom, there is a possibility that
she contracted an STD.

Above all, Cassie and I discussed her situation openly and
honestly. Had her own doctor been honest with her from
the beginning, she would still be his patient. Most impor-

tantly, had she been educated about how to read a lab report and been privy to her own records, she would have known about her minor problem years earlier. She was fortunate it didn't develop into something more serious.

3. Learn to use the report to determine whether the sample was taken properly.

The Pap test lab report may also be called a cytology (study of the cell) report. Since a Pap test is only as reliable as the cell sample on which it is based, the report will describe the quality of the smear taken by your gynecologist. Remember, I said the smear should include both cells from the ectocervix (the outside of the cervix), as well as the endocervical (inner cervical) canal. Naturally, the part of the cervix that a gynecologist taking a sample is most likely to miss would be the hardest place to reach: the endocervical canal. Therefore, look for a statement in the report saying that endocervical cells were present in the sample. Here are a few ways this might be stated:

- Smear quality: endocervical elements present
- Endocervicals: endocervical cells are present
- Endocervicals: glandular cells are present

Another way of evaluating the quality of the specimen taken will sometimes be found under the heading of "smear quality." The laboratory will use words such as "satisfactory or optimal specimen" when a proper sample was taken. Words such as "sub-optimal" or "unsatisfactory" should alert your gynecologist to the necessity of repeating the Pap smear.

- Smear quality: satisfactory or optimal specimen
- Smear quality: sub-optimal or unsatisfactory specimen

By the way, the Pap smear of a woman who has had a hysterectomy (removal of the uterus) will not include ectocervical or endocervical cells, but rather those cells in the area where the cervix (neck of the uterus) used to be.

The Pap smear will allow your gynecologist to identify abnormal cells in the region formerly occupied by the cervix. (This area is called the vaginal cuff.)

4. Learn certain key words that will give you an understanding of the pathologist's diagnosis.

If you've been going to a gynecologist for a while, you may be familiar with a now-outmoded system of labeling Pap smears by classes: Class I, II, III, and so on. Doctors are now coming to realize that using descriptive words—rather than a I, II, III designation—gives them and their patients a lot more information about the condition of the cells being analyzed. If your doctor's lab uses classes (Class I, II, etc.) as the only descriptor of your Pap smear, your gynecologist has the obligation to explain where and how your Pap smear fits in the new, more descriptive classification of Pap smears.

The following outline will help you correlate the new classification with the old.

CLASS (old classification)	DESCRIPTION (new classification)
I	normal; no atypical cells
II	atypical cells: inflammatory atypia or mild dysplasia (CIN I*)
III	suspicious cells: moderate dysplasia (CIN II), severe dysplasia (CIN III)
IV	malignant cells present

The advantage of the new classification is that the Pap smear will alert your gynecologist and you to certain conditions that are the probable cause of your abnormal Pap smear.

---

* See list of terms on page 111.

The following terms may show up on your Pap smear report:

ACTINOMYCES – bacteria found in IUD users; may cause pelvic inflammatory disease (PID)

ATROPHIC – lacking estrogen; usually occurs in menopause

ATYPICAL (OR INFLAMMATORY ATYPIA) – abnormal; usually caused by inflammation

CANDIDA – a yeast infection (*see* Chapter 13)

CARCINOMA IN SITU – an early form of cervical cancer (*see* Chapters 1 and 8)

CHLAMYDIA – a sexually transmitted disease (*see* Chapter 7)

CIN (CERVICAL INTRAEPITHELEAL NEOPLASIA) – dysplasia (*see* Chapters 1 and 8)

CONDYLOMA – another word for HPV (*see* Chapters 1 and 8)

DYSPLASIA – precancerous cells (*see* Chapters 1 and 8)

GARDNERELLA (CLUE CELLS, HAEMOPHILUS) – a type of sexually transmitted vaginal infection (*see* Chapter 13)

HERPES – a sexually transmitted disease (*see* Chapter 10)

HUMAN PAPILLOMA VIRUS (HPV) – a sexually transmitted virus (*see* Chapters 1 and 8)

KOILOCYTOSIS – cells that are infected with HPV (*see* Chapters 1 and 8)

TRICHOMONIASIS a sexually transmitted disease (*see* Chapter 13)

Following are two typical examples of Pap smear reports: first, a normal Pap; second, an abnormal Pap.

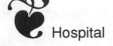

Hospital   Path No: P-92-11649
                Patient:

Med Rec #: (5021)0467-29-99-12   Hosp #: 000-0145729
Date received: 27JAN93   Age: 31 YRS Sex: F
Report Printed: 4FEB93   Location:

Doctor:

CYTOLOGY REPORT

CLINICAL INFORMATION

SPECIMEN TAKEN: 1-27-93
SOURCE: CERVICAL/ENDOCERVICAL SMEAR
LMP: 1-14-93
CLINICAL HISTORY:

CYTOLOGIC DIAGNOSIS:

NO ATYPICAL CELLS PRESENT,
WITHIN NORMAL LIMITS.

ENDOCERVICAL CELLS ARE PRESENT.

INFLAMMATION:

MINIMAL INFLAMMATION PRESENT.

SMEAR QUALITY:

SPECIMEN ADEQUACY IS SATISFACTORY.
        Reported: 02/03/93
        Performed by: cvp
                Verified by:
                        (electronically signed)

Figure 1
Normal Pap smear report

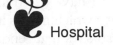 Hospital   Path No: P-92-11649
                                Patient:

Med Rec #: (5021)0467-29-99-12   Hosp #: 000-0145729
Date received: 27JAN93   Age: 31 YRS   Sex: F
Report Printed: 4FEB93   Location:

Doctor:

CYTOLOGY REPORT

CLINICAL INFORMATION

SPECIMEN TAKEN: 1-27-93
SOURCE: CERVICAL/ENDOCERVICAL SMEAR
LMP: 1-14-93
CLINICAL HISTORY:

CYTOLOGIC DIAGNOSIS:

DYSPLASIA: CHANGES SUGGESTIVE OF HPV

ENDOCERVICAL CELLS PRESENT

INFLAMMATION:

SEVERE INFLAMMATION PRESENT.

SMEAR QUALITY:

SPECIMEN ADEQUACY IS SATISFACTORY.
        Reported: 02/03/93
        Performed by: cvp
                Verified by:
                        (electronically signed)

Figure 2
Abnormal Pap smear report

As you look at the first Pap smear report (Figure 1), you will notice that none of the key words I have listed are present. It says "no atypical cells present," which means it's a normal, or negative, Pap smear. It also says that "endo-cervical cells are present," indicating that it is an adequate, or properly taken, sample. There is "minimal inflammation," which is a normal occurrence. The laboratory finishes by re-assuring you that the "specimen is satisfactory." This Pap smear has met all the criteria I have outlined.

Looking at the second Pap smear report (Figure 2), we no-tice the word "dysplasia," which means precancerous cells. It tells us there are "changes suggestive of HPV," alerting you and your doctor that the most likely reason for this dysplasia is the human papilloma virus. As you know by now, this is a sexually transmitted disease; unless your partner is also checked, the likelihood of another abnormal Pap smear in the future is greatly increased. The Pap smear goes on to tell us that "endocervical cells are present" and the specimen ade-quacy is "satisfactory," reassuring us that the Pap smear was properly taken. The "severe inflammation" noted on the Pap smear correlates with the dysplasia caused by the HPV.

If you read a Pap smear correctly, the information is less likely to scare you and should not confuse you. Your doctor should be happy to explain your test results.

With the information I have given you, you now have a simple guide to asking the proper questions of your doctor. This is not intended to make you an expert on interpreting your Pap smear results, rather, it serves as a helpful tool to establish better communication with your doctor. Remem-ber that abnormal cells on a Pap smear do not "just happen." There's a reason, a cure, and a prevention (there's a cure for most of these conditions). Do not accept a report that uses only Class I, II, III, etc., as a description. Instead, insist on a proper explanation of what those abnormal cells in your Pap smear report really mean.

PART THREE

CHAPTER 5

What's an STD?
What's It to Me?

*A must-read if you have ever had sex,
if you are sexually active now, or if you
are about to have sex for the first time*

Picture yourself out for the evening at a social function, surrounded by a lot of people—perhaps at a dance or in a crowded restaurant. You're having a good time, when people around you start coughing and sneezing. You can't see the little droplets full of bacteria and viruses that are now floating in the air, but you know they're there. Just the thought of breathing in all those germs offends you, so you tell your date you want to leave. It's such a relief to get out into the fresh air!

The two of you go home, one thing leads to another and you begin to make love. Now picture yourself in bed having the most intimate physical contact that you can ever have with another person. You are on the pill, so you feel pretty secure that you're not going to get pregnant. But are you safe?

You probably aren't giving a second thought to the body fluids—semen, vaginal fluid, saliva—that you are exchanging with this person. Yet the consequences of sexual contact are far more dangerous than the cold you were afraid of catching earlier. Some of these fluids—and in certain cases the intimate skin-to-skin contact you are having—could transmit diseases that could kill you, make you infertile, affect the health of your future babies, and force you to spend thousands of dollars for gynecological treatment.

One out of four women between the ages of fifteen and fifty-five will contract one or more of these sexually transmitted diseases (STDs), so the odds are that at some point, an STD will touch your life or that of a loved one. This year alone, some twelve million Americans will be diagnosed with an STD; tragically, many well-intentioned but misguided doctors will hide the truth from these patients—that their afflictions were sexually transmitted. Countless other infected people will go undiagnosed, unaware of the internal damage an STD is doing to them, while they unintentionally pass the disease to their sexual partners. With the exception of AIDS, many people have never even heard of some of the deadliest STDs, or mistakenly think that only extremely promiscuous people, drug addicts, or prostitutes and their clients ever get these diseases. No wonder STDs have been called the "silent epidemic."

> What impact has the AIDS epidemic had on people becoming informed about other sexually transmitted diseases? Initially, I think, when people thought about AIDS patients, they told themselves, "This will never happen to me. It's somebody else's problem." Now we're starting to make progress in talking about issues of sexual communication. What we haven't yet done as a culture is to talk specifically about the other sexually transmitted diseases that have been overshadowed by AIDS.
>
> —Peggy Clarke, executive director,
> American Social Health Association (ASHA)

What are sexually transmitted diseases?

Did you know that a large percentage of disorders that gynecologists diagnose are contracted sexually? For example, are you aware that dysplasia (abnormal development, or growth, of cells) is a sexually transmitted condition and that cervical cancer is a sexually transmitted disease? Did you know that if you have chronic "pelvic pain" or "a pelvic infection," you very likely have pelvic inflammatory disease (PID), which is transmitted sexually?

When you hear of sexually transmitted disease, do you think solely of AIDS, or of what used to be termed venereal diseases—syphilis, gonorrhea ("the clap"), or herpes? With AIDS making daily headlines, other STDs threatening women's lives and fertility aren't as well known.

Do you assume that other STDs are nuisance infections? Other than AIDS, the top three threats to women's sexual health in the 1990s are chlamydia, condyloma (also known as genital warts—the human papilloma virus, or HPV), and gonorrhea. In all, some twenty-five diseases are spread through sexual contact. Most of the widespread STDs—chlamydia, condyloma, hepatitis B, etc.—are deadly if not caught in time. The good news is, the majority are curable and all are preventable.

How can I get a sexually transmitted disease?

Does the answer to this question seem obvious? Well, you'd be surprised at the myths that still prevail about sexually transmitted disease. You get an STD by having intercourse—vaginal, oral, or anal—with an infected person. Some STDs are spread through contact with body fluids, especially semen, vaginal fluids, and blood. A few STDs can also be transmitted via direct contact with infected skin. The common denominator, however, is the intimate contact of sex. As more women have sex with more partners, their chances of contracting an STD escalate. Have you ever really thought about that warning you hear so often: women sleep not only with their partners; they also sleep with every person their partner has ever slept with.

Here are some of the most frequent questions patients ask me about the transmission of STDs:

Can you catch an STD in a swimming pool or by using the same bathroom facilities as somebody who is infected?
This may sound flippant, but the only way you could catch an STD in a swimming pool or a bathroom is by having sex with an infected person in a pool or a bathroom.

Can you catch an STD from sharing an infected person's towel or clothing?
The chances of this happening are so small that I have never—in my many years of gynecological practice—seen a patient who contracted an STD this way.

Can you get an STD from kissing?
Very, very rarely.

Can you catch an STD by using an infected person's eating utensils or drinking glass, or sharing their food?
No.

Do birth control pills protect a woman from catching an STD?
No.

Can you catch an STD from someone the first time you ever have sex?

Yes. The bacteria and viruses that cause STDs are just as infectious whether you are having sex for the first time—even on your wedding night—or the umpteenth time. It only takes one act of sex for someone to transmit an STD to you.

I heard that STDs are easy to spot on a man and that they always show up right away in males. Is this true?

No. Most STDs cause few or no symptoms in males. A man could infect you with an STD without ever knowing he had the disease.

Do gynecologists routinely test patients for all the most dangerous STDs?

I confess to planting this last question to make an important point. Standard tests for STDs are not included with a routine exam and Pap smear unless specifically requested by the patient.

By far the most prevalent and dangerous myth about catching STDs is that only "bad" women run the risk of getting them. Many times, after I have broken the news to a patient that she has an STD, she will voice feelings like these:

"How could this have happened to me, when I have never been promiscuous? I only have one relationship at a time!"

"There has to be some mistake! I thought only prostitutes caught those diseases."

Actually, I do have call girls in my practice, none of whom are IV drug users, and these women seldom catch any kind of STD. Why not? They are streetwise; their livelihood depends on their sexual health. These professionals could rival a doctor in their skill at spotting an STD in a male partner, and of course they insist on using condoms. They visit the gynecologist every three to four months, asking to be tested for every STD in the book, and are unabashed at informing the doctor about their sexual behavior. When they do need treatment for an STD, they follow through completely; and if they have four or five partners, they see that their partners get treated and their partners' partners. Most of all, they understand the risks and take precautions to avoid them.

More often than not, victims of the silent epidemic are otherwise intelligent women who haven't taken the responsibility to educate themselves, because if they think about STDs at all, they still believe that "those" diseases only happen to "those" women.

Now, I would never advocate that you become streetwise in the same fashion as my patients who are call girls. You may not choose to do what they do, but perhaps you should know what they know about STDs. For example, they know the symptoms that should bring a woman to her doctor to be checked for STDs.

What are the symptoms of STDs in women?

Here's a brief summary of warning signs that may alert your doctor to the presence of a sexually transmitted disease. (By the way, it's a myth that if symptoms go away on their own, you're cured. If you have an STD, its symptoms may appear and disappear, but the disease remains and—unless treated—usually becomes more serious.)

- Abnormal Pap smear
- Lower back pain
- Burning or pain during urination

- Fever
- Pain resembling menstrual cramps
- Pain during intercourse
- Pelvic or abdominal pain
- Sores, bumps, or blisters in genital or anal area, or around mouth
- Spotting between periods
- Swelling in genital area
- Swelling or redness in throat
- Unusual vaginal odor
- Unusually frequent urination
- Vaginal discharge
- Vaginal itching or burning

What are the symptoms of STDs in men?

- Burning or pain during urination (men seldom get urinary infections that aren't related to STDs)
- Discharge from penis
- Itching or burning in genital area
- Pain in testicles
- Redness in genital area
- Sores, bumps, or blisters in genital or anal area or around mouth

What are the physical dangers if I get an STD?

Chapter 1 addressed the most serious health risks involved in being sexually active; Chapters 6 through 14 will go into more detail about the risks and consequences associated with sexually transmitted diseases. Following is a summary of the physical dangers that STDs pose to women and to children born to infected women.

Risks and/or consequences to women:

- Bartholin gland abscess
- Blindness
- Cancer of the liver
- Cancer of the vagina
- Cancer of the vulva
- Chronic fatigue
- Chronic pelvic pain
- Cirrhosis of the liver or permanent liver damage
- Cancer of the cervix
- Death from rupture of a tubal pregnancy, rupture of an abscess, or AIDS
- Dysplasia (precancerous cells)
- Heart disease
- Hysterectomy or partial hysterectomy
- Infertility or reduced fertility due to scarring of the reproductive organs
- Insanity
- Nervous disorders
- Oophorectomy (removal of the ovaries), causing early menopause
- Stroke

Risks and/or consequences to newborns:

- Anemia and other blood disorders
- Blindness
- Bone or dental deformities
- Brain damage
- Early death
- Eye inflammation
- Infection of throat
- Infections of ears and respiratory system
- Infections of vagina and rectum
- Low birth weight

- Pneumonia
- Premature birth
- Stillbirth

What are the emotional consequences if I get an STD?

Throughout the years that I have been a practicing gynecologist, not a day has gone by when a patient doesn't feel a wide range of emotions after being told she has a sexually transmitted disease. I'm not speaking now about the medical consequences of having an STD; rather, I'm talking about deep feelings like shame, mortification, guilt, and self-loathing that emerge when a woman learns she has one of "those" diseases. No matter how well my patients anticipate that they would handle such news, when it hits them personally, it hits them hard.

On the heels of these feelings come overwhelming anxieties. Many patients fear that no one will ever want to date them or get close to them again. Others fear they will never bear children. The impact of being diagnosed with an STD can stay with a woman for years, long after the disease has been cured or brought under control.

A number of people who call the National STD Hotline are very concerned, angry, hostile, fearful, depressed, and in mourning. Most are grieving the loss of something. They may be recognizing that they've lost their ability to reproduce; they may be mourning the death of their partner to a sexually transmitted disease. But what all the calls have in common is that they reflect our society's main problems relating to these diseases: poor communication and a lack of information about STDs.

—Peggy Clarke, executive director, ASHA

How does my doctor find out if I have an STD?

Don't assume that your gynecologist will automatically test you for STDs or even bring up the topic. In my opinion, all gynecologists should educate patients about STDs and advise sexually active patients to undergo testing. Unfortunately, this just isn't routine procedure at the present time. It may be up to you to request that you be tested. If necessary, demand to be tested. If you are diagnosed with an STD, what you will gain through early detection and treatment will far outweigh the extra cost of the tests.

Most STD tests are simple office procedures, including visual inspection, the Pap smear, doing a culture (taking a small sample from an area thought to be infected and "growing" it in a lab), and running blood tests.

Having yourself tested and treated will accomplish nothing unless your partner does the same. Otherwise, he will reinfect you, and the two of you may transmit the infection back and forth as if it were a ping-pong ball. He can be tested by a urologist, a general practitioner, or a health clinic professional.

Frequently a patient will tell me, "I'm sure my partner got checked for STDs, because he had a physical with a blood test and that tests for everything." Wrong! A man's routine physical does not check for sexually transmitted diseases; most STDs cannot be detected by a simple blood test. Just like you, your partner needs to specifically request that he be tested for STDs.

How are STDs treated?

Fortunately, the majority of STDs are easily treated if detected early. Some STDs cannot be cured, but in most cases treatment can prevent further damage. Often, an inexpensive dose of antibiotics is the only treatment necessary. Chapters 6 through 14 will describe treatment methods for each of the most common STDs. Surgical and other procedures commonly used in the diagnosis and treatment of some STDs will be described in Chapter 16.

How can STDs be prevented?

Please read Chapter 17, which is devoted to this important topic. I will explain why there is no such thing as "safe sex." After all, the only person you can be 100 percent sure of is you. Even if you have only one partner and he is absolutely faithful to you, he may—without knowing it—be carrying an STD that he acquired long before he met you. You can, however, have "safer sex" if you educate yourself and take the precautions that will be discussed. If you choose your partners wisely, limit the number of partners you have, are prudent in your choice of sexual practices, use condoms correctly during every sexual act, and ensure that you and your partner are tested regularly, you have a good chance of remaining free of STDs.

In the following nine chapters, I have used a simple question and answer format to brief you on the most common STDs. These chapters are intended to arm you with the facts you need so that you and your doctor can work together toward safeguarding your health.

CHAPTER 6

AIDS and HIV:
Still Confused?

*Heterosexual women are
now at greatest risk*

Key words:

AIDS, HIV, Acquired Immune Deficiency Syndrome

Risks and/or consequences:

- Enlarged lymph nodes
- Weight loss
- Pneumonia
- Cancer
- Death

Charlotte had one special relationship in college. After graduation, she and her boyfriend went their separate ways. She got a job in the city and began to date a new man. That relationship lasted two years. Recently, she went to her gynecologist for a routine checkup and Pap test. As an afterthought, she requested an HIV test, explaining that she was back on the dating scene and wanted to be able to reassure any future partners. A few days later, her doctor phoned to say that the lab might have made an error and could she please come back in to repeat some of the tests. Much to her dismay, she found out that it was the HIV test her doctor wanted to repeat; her original test had come back positive. When the second test also showed her positive for HIV, her life as she knew it would never be the same.

After the initial shock wore off, she felt numb, but through the numbness one question emerged: She was not a drug user and had not been promiscuous, so how in the world had she gotten infected? She learned the answer when, at her doctor's urging, she contacted her previous partners to notify them that she was HIV-positive. When she alerted her most recent partner, he tested negative for HIV. But he had to live through six months of fear before a second test also showed him negative. The man who had been her lover in college was in the advanced stages of AIDS. He confessed that he had experimented with IV drugs while in high school.

Today Charlotte lives in limbo. She still feels fine and as yet has not developed any signs of AIDS. Yet she can see no future, no marriage or children. She feels that there is nothing in front of her but bleakness—waiting to die. Her only hope is that a cure is found in time.

What is it?

AIDS (acquired immune deficiency syndrome) is a viral infection caused by the human immunodeficiency virus (HIV). This virus is selective in that it chooses to attack the immune system cells within the body. Once HIV begins its spread throughout these cells, it destroys them, causing a multitude of illnesses. The World Health Organization estimates that by the year 2000, forty million adults and children will have HIV, and women will comprise over half of these patients. About 100,000 HIV infections resulting from heterosexual sex have been reported in the United States since 1985. Heterosexual sex accounts for 75 percent of AIDS cases worldwide.

How can I get it?

AIDS is spread by the transmission of infected fluids from one person to another. The virus is found in semen, menstrual blood, vaginal discharge, tears, blood, urine, stools, and even breast milk. The amount of virus present in a body fluid determines the likelihood of that fluid infecting a person.

The most common way HIV is transmitted is by sexual intercourse, due to the high concentration of the HIV virus in semen and the likelihood of repetitive exposure to the virus. It is presumed that the body may be able to fight off small concentrations of the virus found in fluids such as tears or saliva, but unable to defend itself against the larger amounts usually found in blood or semen.

The second largest group of patients with AIDS encompasses those who were infected through blood transmissions. Included in this group are IV drug users who have shared contaminated needles, and recipients of blood transfusions (especially those prior to 1985, when routine screening of blood for HIV became standard). Babies are also infected by the blood they receive through the mother's placenta. This can happen either during pregnancy or delivery. Less commonly, contamination can occur when health care workers accidentally stick themselves with contaminated needles or handle infected tissue or debris in an unsafe manner.

AIDS is not transmitted through casual contact. Fortunately, it has been shown that the virus cannot survive long in the open air. There is no evidence you can get AIDS by kissing, hugging, sharing bathroom facilities, or sharing drinking glasses or food.

In short, you must realize that your main risk comes from sexual intercourse. The myth that gay men and prostitutes are the only ones susceptible to the disease is just that—a myth. The gay community is actively implementing sexual education, and we are now beginning to see an actual decline in the number of AIDS cases in homosexual men. Sadly, the number of HIV-positive women is increasing at a staggering rate.

I hope I am not scaring you, but I do want to warn you. If you think that AIDS could not happen to you and that it only happens to "other people," you are dead wrong. Look at Magic Johnson: superstar, athlete, healthy family man. He did not use IV drugs, he did not engage in homosexual activities—but he practiced unsafe sex. No one is a match for this virus.

What are the symptoms?

Many of you already spend countless hours worrying over whether or not you are infected with AIDS. Until routine HIV testing becomes commonplace, knowing the symptoms will help to alleviate fear and increase our understanding of this complicated disease.

Once the symptoms appear—which can be years after the initial transmission of the virus—they begin as mildly as weight loss, swollen glands (lymph nodes), lack of appetite, gastrointestinal disorders such as constipation or diarrhea, fever, skin rashes, and progressive weakness. AIDS symptoms can resemble those of other diseases. The difference is, AIDS symptoms don't go away; on the contrary, they progress with unpredictable speed. Some patients with these symptoms do not develop full-blown AIDS right away. A person who has tested HIV-positive and is thus able to transmit the disease may appear healthy and vital for many years.

Once the immune system is destroyed or sufficiently impaired, certain infections that would usually not infect a healthy patient take over. These are called "opportunistic" infections and include pneumocystis pneumonia (which appears in 64 percent of AIDS patients), and candidiasis, a fungus infection attacking the esophagus and lungs (which appears in 9 percent of AIDS patients). Vaginal candidiasis, or yeast infection, is not an AIDS infection.

Other, less common, AIDS-associated infections include cryptococcosis (systemic yeast infection), histoplasmosis (parasitic infection), and cytomegalovirus (infections caused by virus). All these mimic each other by producing pneumonia or diarrhea, making the symptoms a puzzle for both doctor and patient. Two cancers are included in the Centers for Disease Control's (CDC) definition of AIDS: Kaposi's sarcoma (malignancy of the blood vessels) and lymphoma (malignancy of lymphoid tissue). However, these are rare in women infected heterosexually. The CDC is presently revising the definition of AIDS to include all diseases whose association with HIV is becoming clearer.

Within a year of development of these AIDS symptoms, 50 percent of the patients die; after three years, 90 percent die. We still do not understand the timing of the disease. We do know that 65 percent of women who die of AIDS were not properly diagnosed prior to death. Remember that the medical profession is sometimes influenced by the same myths and taboos as the rest of society.

What are the dangers if I get it?

People who are HIV-positive may appear and feel healthy, but the majority will unfortunately develop full-blown AIDS with all the horrible symptoms of the disease. Tragically, death is the final outcome. The same dangers apply to your sexual partner and to your unborn child.

How does my doctor find out if I have it?

Reality tells me that the major problem you will face is reluctance on the part of your doctor to discuss this subject with you. Therefore, take control and demand testing. If you are worried, suspicious, or scared, don't let that stop you from being tested.

Once you've decided to be tested, your doctor will perform a simple blood test. The test used for screening is called ELISA (enzyme-linked immunosorbent assay), and will usually detect HIV within six months of exposure. Sometimes the test will come back positive due to lab error, so a diagnosis of HIV is not made on the first positive test. If the ELISA test is positive twice, a more sensitive blood test called Western Blot is performed. If this test is positive, the patient is determined to be infected with HIV. These tests are quick and easy and are usually performed in your doctor's office.

If you have been exposed to the virus, it takes from two weeks to six months before the body produces enough antibodies to produce a positive ELISA test. Therefore, if you are concerned about exposure within the last six months, you should be tested twice: once two months after the suspected exposure, and a second time six months after the suspected exposure. If you and your partner have been monogamous for those six months and both test negative, it is fairly safe to assume your relationship is HIV-negative. Free testing is available in most major cities through your health department.

How is it treated?

There is no cure for AIDS, but there is now more hope than ever. Every day we read about new drugs and treatments for AIDS patients (such as AZT). Worldwide, people are putting their mental energies and resources into finding a cure, and prolonging and improving the lives of patients with the disease. The longer we keep patients with HIV from developing AIDS, the better their chances are of being alive for that cure.

Researchers are striving toward multiple goals. One is to find a cure that would destroy the AIDS virus and restore the immune system to its normal state. Another is to develop drugs that would block the effect of the virus and keep the disease under control. A third objective is to develop medicines that would control or cure those opportunistic diseases associated with HIV. The ultimate mission is to develop a vaccine that would prevent infection. Staying healthy by exercising and eating a proper diet goes a long way in delaying an HIV patient from developing AIDS and ultimately helps in the treatment of the disease.

How can I prevent it?

Prevention begins with being informed. Not a day goes by in my practice in which I don't hear "I'm embarrassed to ask him," "He won't wear a condom," or "It takes away from spontaneity." Not one of these is a valid excuse to allow yourself and others to die from sex. You must take an active role in preventing the spread of this disease. If your partner finds discussing previous partners, sexual practices, use of condoms, or history of drug use annoying, I strongly suggest you reevaluate your relationship. It is far more uncomfortable to die from AIDS than it is to approach this issue with your partner.

Choose your partner wisely. Limit your number of sexual partners. Know if he is or has been bisexual, an IV drug user, or promiscuous; know if he has had other sexually transmitted diseases (STDs) in the past or if he has been a recipient of a blood transfusion. Remember that if he answers no, your next question should be "What about the history of your previous partners?"

Obviously, this can become a nightmare. To simplify the problem, you should always use a latex condom during any sexual act, including oral sex. It is important for you to understand that condoms make sex safer—not safe. Condoms can break or be used inappropriately. Spermicides have not been shown to kill the HIV virus but may act as additional protection when used with condoms.

In this age, starting a sexual relationship should involve knowledge of STDs (including AIDS), testing for STDs (including AIDS), selecting the proper condoms, and maintaining a mutually monogamous relationship. Peace of mind will definitely outweigh these minor inconveniences.

CHAPTER 7

Chlamydia:
The Most Silent STD

*The most prevalent STD linked
to pelvic disease and infertility*

Key words:

Endometritis, Salpingitis, Pelvic Inflammatory Disease
(PID), Cervicitis, Urethritis, Prostatitis

Risks and/or consequences:

- Chronic abdominal and pelvic pain
- Infertility
- Tubal (ectopic) pregnancy
- Hysterectomy
- Bartholin gland abscess

After three years of marriage, Debby and her husband
Charles wanted to start a family. When Debby still had not
conceived after six months, she sought her gynecologist's
help. When he performed a laparoscopy, he found extensive adhesions blocking Debby's fallopian tubes. He removed as much of the scar tissue as possible. With renewed

hope, the couple tried for another six months to conceive without success.

Although Debby's gynecologist suggested further surgery, she felt she needed a better understanding of her options. She read up on infertility and finally consulted an infertility specialist for a second opinion. After reviewing her records, he asked about each partner's sexual history. He also screened her for sexually transmitted diseases (STDs).

Much to Debby's surprise, one culture came back positive. An STD she had never heard of called chlamydia turned out to be the culprit behind her infertility. Sadly, she learned that she or Charles could have contracted chlamydia years before, and neither would have known they were infected.

The infertility specialist treated both partners so that the chlamydia wouldn't do more damage, but Debby still faces further surgery to attempt to restore her fertility. Even with treatment, there is no guarantee she will ever bear a child.

Adding to the emotional anguish is the knowledge that all this could have been prevented if Debby's gynecologist had done routine screening for STDs during her yearly exams. When she called her gynecologist to ask why he hadn't tested her for chlamydia, he answered, "I thought you were a nice girl. It never dawned on me to test you."

What is it?

The most common STD in the United States, chlamydia, is a bacterial disease caused by the organism *Chlamydia trachomatis*. It is estimated that between four and five million new cases occur each year, but this is a very conservative estimate. Most states do not require physicians to report this disease to public health officials. As recently as 1990, while giving a seminar to the nurses of the Dallas Public

Health Department, I was dismayed to learn that due to lack of funds, the department was not even testing for chlamydia.

In 1986 Congress allocated only $4.5 million for chlamydia control. This is less than one dollar per patient. This figure shrinks even further in the overall picture, considering that in 1990 chlamydia required an estimated $2 billion in health care costs.

Chlamydia is known as the "silent epidemic": silent because of its vague symptoms, and because no one—including our public health departments—pays it much notice; and epidemic because of the staggering number of cases that are recorded each year.

How can I get it?

A chlamydial infection is contracted through sexual intercourse. You cannot get it from towels or toilet seats. It only takes one sexual encounter with an infected partner to acquire the disease. Obviously, the more partners you have, the higher your risk will be. But the idea that you have to be promiscuous to develop an STD such as chlamydia is totally false.

What are the symptoms in women?

Most women exposed to chlamydia have no symptoms. Those who do experience warning signs will notice a wide range of complaints. A slight increase in vaginal secretions may be present; this presents itself as a watery mucous-like secretion, (which may cause vaginal irritation such as redness, burning, or itching). Frequent and painful urination is present in most cases. Abnormalities in bleeding patterns during a menstrual cycle are common, such as excessive flow, spotting between cycles, and increased cramping.

A woman may also experience spotting or bleeding after sexual intercourse. Persistent painful intercourse is another warning sign. This pain will resemble a cramping or aching sensation in your lower abdomen or pelvis. Contrary to what you may have been told in the past, this type of discomfort is not normal. Ask yourself this question: If it didn't hurt before, why is it hurting now? Chlamydia may be the answer.

What are the symptoms in men?

In men, chlamydia symptoms occur in the urethra, the thin tube that runs through the penis carrying urine from the bladder. When a chlamydial infection settles in the urethra, it causes painful urination and the feeling of needing to urinate frequently. A man may also have a clear or pale yellow penile discharge. This will be a watery discharge as opposed to the thick discharge of gonorrhea.

Remember that men do not usually get bladder infections. If your partner has urinary complaints, this should be a warning signal. Chlamydia, if untreated, can lead to epididymitis, an inflammation of the testicles that can cause sterility.

What are the dangers if I get it?

It is staggering to me that a disease that can be treated so simply and so inexpensively (with one round of antibiotics) can also cause such devastating results. To help you understand the severity of the problem, I will take you through the most relevant dangers or complications that can be caused by a chlamydial infection.

Chlamydia can cause an infection in the cervix called cervicitis. This can be one of the many causes of an abnormal pap smear. As the outer cells in the cervix become infected, they produce a pus-like substance that becomes mixed with the vaginal mucous. The resulting persistent discharge is frequently misdiagnosed as a yeast infection. It is impossible for a woman to determine whether she has chlamydia by merely looking at her discharge.

If the patient goes untreated, the infection will affect the uterus, the fallopian tubes, and ovaries, producing a serious condition known as pelvic inflammatory disease (PID). Over 400,000 women are hospitalized annually for PID, and despite aggressive treatment in the hospital with intravenous antibiotics and /or surgeries, the reproductive organs are not always left unscathed.

As these organs become involved, the dangers of the disease become more evident. Scars (adhesions) damage the fallopian tubes, making them prone to tubal pregnancies (ectopics). This means that the pregnancy develops in the fallopian tubes instead of in the uterus. Potentially life-threatening, this condition is responsible for at least 10 to 15 percent of maternal deaths.

The scars can completely block the fallopian tubes, rendering a woman sterile. An estimated 40 to 50 percent of all visits to an infertility specialist could have been prevented by routine chlamydial screening.

When a woman with a chlamydial infection is fortunate enough to become pregnant, she still runs a higher risk of miscarriage and stillborns. If she delivers the baby through the vaginal canal, the baby has a high risk of developing an eye infection called conjunctivitis, which could ultimately lead to blindness. The baby can also get pneumonia from the chlamydial infection.

Chlamydia also creates glue-like adhesions that make the ovaries and fallopian tubes stick to themselves and to other surrounding organs. This creates pelvic pain and pain during intercourse, usually necessitating surgical procedures to alleviate the discomfort. A large number of gynecological procedures (such as laparoscopies and hysterectomies) are the direct consequence of an untreated chlamydial infection.

Another consequence of chlamydia that we see often is an abscess of the Bartholin gland, a small lubricating gland located at the opening to the vagina. Chlamydia can cause this gland to become infected; it swells up and is extremely painful. To treat this, your doctor will lance and drain the abscess and put you on antibiotics. If the abscess returns—which frequently happens—your doctor will need to deeply clean out the gland. This operation is called marsupialization and requires a general anesthetic.

How does my doctor find out if I have it?

Keeping in mind that the average cost of infertility treatment runs into the thousands of dollars—and that most insurance companies will not pay for it—and bearing in mind that chlamydia testing is not a routine part of a yearly examination, you must demand that your doctor perform this simple test so you can avoid not only going broke but becoming sterile.

Testing for chlamydia is simple and relatively painless. During your pelvic examination, the doctor will scrape some cells from within the cervix to retrieve a sample. The method the laboratory will use for analyzing the sample varies from a culture (Chlamydiazime), in which the bacteria actually grow on a culture dish, to a special immunofluorescence test (Microtrac), where the bacteria are identified via microscope. These tests take an average of two to four days to yield results, and the price ranges from $60 to $100. Your doctor can also opt for office tests in which the result is available in thirty minutes, and the cost is far less expensive.

Unfortunately, the tests are not 100 percent accurate. A woman whose lab results were negative could still have chlamydia. Thus, when a woman undergoes a pelvic exam, it is important that she tell her doctor if she experiences pain or discomfort. Sometimes this is the only clue the doctor will have to suspect chlamydia, and he usually will choose to treat her with antibiotics even prior to the results of the culture. When in doubt, it is better to treat a patient with $20 worth of antibiotics than to wonder whether or not the laboratory failed to detect chlamydia.

How is it treated?

The one happy aspect of this story is that chlamydia is easily cured. Usually a seven- to ten-day course of antibiotics (such as tetracycline, doxycycline, or erythromyocin) is all that is required. Newer antibiotics show tremendous promise in treating the disease and require fewer days of antibiotic therapy.

Keep in mind that your partner must be treated simultaneously. It does not matter whether he has no symptoms or his culture is negative. You must both take the antibiotic to avoid reinfection. Chlamydia is 100 percent curable when both you and your partner follow the proper course of treatment.

This disease does not reoccur on its own. In order for you to experience a reinfection, three things must happen: 1) you did not take the antibiotics properly, 2) your partner did not take the antibiotics properly, and 3) someone else is involved in your relationship. Time and time again I hear in my practice, "I just seem to be susceptible to these infections." As noted in prior chapters, women are not "susceptible" to infections such as chlamydia. They are always brought into the relationship; they do not just happen.

How can I prevent it?

Besides following the advice that condoms (and not diamonds) are a girl's best friend, you can prevent chlamydia by limiting your number of sexual partners and by undergoing routine testing. The best ounce of prevention is in making your partner a true partner in your relationship. Demand that he gets tested and/or treated. Make him understand that his lack of symptoms does not prove absence of the disease. Your gynecologist should not only educate you regarding chlamydia but should also be willing to discuss it with your partner if you so desire.

I know talking about these things is not easy in a relationship, but neither is discussing infertility or hysterectomy. Part of the role of a gynecologist is to counsel, advise, and educate her patients on sexual issues. A gynecologist has a responsibility to your sexual health. That is why you confer with us about personal issues such as birth control, pain during sex, and spotting after sex. Discussing ways to prevent STDs is no different. Use us as a resource. Doctors will tell you things that mom never did.

CHAPTER 8

Genital Warts: A Major Cause of Cervical Cancer

An abnormal Pap smear may be the first warning sign

Key words:

Condyloma, Human Papilloma Virus (HPV), Dysplasia, Koilocytotic Atypia

Risks and/or consequences:

- Dysplasia (precancerous cells)
- Cervical cancer
- Vulvar cancer
- Vaginal cancer
- Anal cancer

Vicky didn't notice the small bump when it first appeared on her vulva. When it enlarged, and even when a few more bumps developed, she thought this was a mild irritation that would probably disappear on its own. When the bumps continued to spread, she went to her gynecologist, and there she learned that she had the human papilloma virus

(HPV). The results of a Pap smear showed that, fortunately, the warts hadn't spread to her cervix.

Vicky's gynecologist was able to reassure her emotionally as well as medically. He helped her realize that she wasn't the only person who ever had HPV and that she had no reason to feel ashamed. He called in her partner to educate him as well and referred him to a urologist for screening.

Treatment began with topically applied chemicals. As sometimes happens, her condition did not not improve after many visits. The warts spread to the point that Vicky had to undergo laser surgery. In the meantime, her partner was found to have a small lesion, and the urologist treated him with cryotherapy to freeze the infected area.

After Vicky and her partner had faithfully used condoms for three months, both were checked and, happily, showed no signs of reinfection. While there is no cure for HPV, the chances are good that with regular checkups, the couple will remain symptom-free.

What is it?

HPV is the fastest growing sexually transmitted disease in the United States. Between twelve and fourteen million women in the United States have HPV. It occurs in sexually active women and men of all ages, races, and social classes, affecting heterosexuals and homosexuals alike. Babies can be infected by their mothers during birth, although this is rare. As doctors are not required to report HPV to public health authorities, we can only estimate that one to two million new cases of HPV are diagnosed each year in the United States.

HPV infections are caused by a group of viruses of which there are over sixty types. HPV types 6, 11, 16, 18, 31, 33, and 35 are the ones that cause cancerous and precancerous changes of the genitalia and can also cause venereal warts.

Experts agree that HPV is a factor in 90 percent of cervical cancer cases and the cell abnormalities that precede them. Many of these experts believe that certain types of HPV are the single most important risk factor in cervical cancer. Cervical cancer is a sexually transmitted disease.

How can I get it?

Genital HPV is most commonly spread through sexual contact with an infected person, whether by vaginal, anal, or oral sex. The biggest problem with HPV is that it can go undetected for a very long time. Recent studies have shown that 35 to 45 percent of otherwise healthy individuals may harbor the virus without developing warts or other abnormalities. Therefore, they may transmit the disease unknowingly. It is clear that a person may be exposed to HPV years prior to showing any signs or symptoms. Developing a genital wart does not necessarily mean your current partner is unfaithful.

What are the symptoms in women?

When venereal warts are visible, they appear as flesh-colored clusters of cauliflower-like growths. They are painless and usually do not bleed. Some patients complain of vulvar itching. These warts are usually found on the vulva, inside the vagina, or around the rectum. Any bump in your genital area should be examined by your gynecologist.

Venereal warts may be so small that patient and doctor will not be able to see them without specialized equipment. When the virus affects the cervix, there are no symptoms. Your first warning of cervical involvement is an abnormal Pap smear. Abnormal Paps indicating dysplasia (precancerous cells), koilocytotic atypia (meaning cells affected by a virus), or condyloma are usually associated with HPV.

There is no such thing as abnormal cells that "just happen." Never accept this explanation from your doctor. You must associate the word "dysplasia" with sexual transmission, and as with every STD, your partner must be examined and treated also. I am saddened by the countless times that I have encountered patients who had multiple procedures, such as lasers of the cervix, but were never told by their physicians that their partners needed treatment.

What are the symptoms in men?

HPV is a sexist disease—men have fewer complications and side effects from this virus. Rarely does a male die as a consequence of condyloma; however, it is not unheard of for this to happen.

The warts can be found on the penis and less commonly on the scrotum and anus. It is much harder for a physician to identify warts on a male. Unfortunately, the lesions can be quite small and escape detection by an untrained eye. Twenty percent of the time the virus targets the urethra, making lesions invisible to the eye and requiring a specially trained doctor, such as a urologist, to identify the virus.

Your partner has not had a proper exam unless the doctor uses special solutions and magnifying equipment for examination of the male genitalia. A comment I frequently hear in my practice is "My partner went to the doctor and he didn't have anything." The proper comment should be "His doctor may not have been able to see any lesions, but he will recheck him in three months."

What are the dangers if I get it?

The primary dangers for women of an HPV infection include cancerous and precancerous lesions of the cervix, vagina, and vulva. Besides the obvious dangers, these conditions have significant emotional consequences. If allowed to progress, these conditions can lead to major and sometimes painful and disfiguring surgeries such as vulvectomies (partial or total removal of the vulva), hysterectomies, laser surgeries, or cone biopsies. Remember, the condition that caused Diane's death (see Introduction) started with a simple HPV infection.

On rare occasions I have seen pregnant women undergo cesarean sections because the untreated venereal warts had grown so large that they blocked the vaginal canal. If a baby is delivered through a vagina infected with venereal warts, it can develop warts (papillomas) on its vocal cords. Again, these instances are rare but they do happen.

If left untreated in the male, HPV can cause penile and anal cancer. I remember a particular patient whose partner had multiple venereal warts on his penis. The urologist had to use lasers to "burn off" the infected areas. Although the warts are gone, the scars left behind make sexual intercourse extremely painful for him.

How does my doctor find out if I have it?

If a woman detects a small wart-like growth on her genitalia, the physician will take a sample (vulvar biopsy) and have it analyzed. The physician may apply a special solution (acetic acid) that can highlight less detectable areas of abnormality. He may also use a special magnifying instrument (colposcope) to be able to see areas having microscopic infection.

If abnormalities have formed on the cervix, a Pap smear will inform you and your doctor of those changes. As you know by now, the Pap smear simply alerts your doctor to problems; it does not necessarily tell him the severity of the problem, which is assessed when a cervical biopsy is done with the aid of the colposcope. Scary as it sounds, the discomfort is minimal and the small piece of tissue (biopsy) is minute; no stitches are required. At most, your doctor will prescribe some minor analgesics. Cervical biopsy patients do not need to take a day off work or make special arrangements to get home. Do not let the word "biopsy" scare you.

How is it treated?

There is no cure for the virus. There is also no oral medicine or shot that can treat HPV. However, there are numerous ways to treat the damage the virus can cause. The goal of treatment is to remove all those lesions that are visible or to remove all those areas of cells in the cervix that are affected by the virus. Some of the most common methods are described below:

- **Podophyllin** or **trichloracetic acid** are caustic agents that are applied to the surface of the warts by a health care provider. These agents cannot be used inside the vagina or if the patient is pregnant. Treatment starts around $30.

- **Podofilox** is a diluted solution of podophyllin and can be used at home with proper instructions. The drug is applied topically and costs around $55.

- **Cryotherapy** (freezing of the affected area) is a simple office procedure used to remove warts on the outside genitalia and abnormal cells in the cervix. The treatment costs $120 to $150.

- **Electrocautery** (electric current) is used in the same manner as cryotherapy. The treatment also costs between $120 and $150.

- **Laser therapy** uses a beam of light to destroy affected areas. This is far more expensive and is reserved for severe cases of dysplasia of the cervix or for vulvar warts too large to treat with simple methods. The cost ranges from $600 up.

- **Cone biopsies** are reserved for extensive or serious HPV infections of the cervix. They require anesthesia and involve the risk of excessive bleeding and/or damage to the cervix, causing sterility. Including hospital and anesthesia bills, costs are around $3,000.

- A new procedure called **LLETZ** (large loop excision of the transformation zone) mimics the cone biopsy, but has been proven to be as, if not more, effective in treating cervical disease due to HPV. Major advantages are that this procedure is performed in the doctor's office with no anesthesia, costs are far less and—most importantly—the damage to the cervix is far less than with a cone biopsy. Most competent gynecologists should know how to perform this new procedure, making the typical cone biopsy almost an obsolete treatment for HPV infections of the cervix. If your doctor does not know how to perform this procedure, ask him to refer you to someone who does. This procedure should cost around $700 to $1,000.

- **Interferon** is an anti-viral drug that is used for patients who do not respond to conventional therapy. It involves a series of injections into the affected areas and may be considered experimental by some authorities. Insurance companies usually do not pay for this procedure. Costs begin at $1,000.

Treatment for HPV usually requires multiple visits to your doctor and is likely to frustrate both partners. Nevertheless,

HPV can be beaten. The battle requires cooperation and coordination between the patient, her gynecologist, the partner, and his urologist. Unless those four people communicate and work together, failure is inevitably the result. The gynecologist should be the party who orchestrates this network.

Even when all the proper things are done, a patient may still have relapses years later. So if your partner says he was treated five years ago and he has been faithful to you for the last five years, it is not naive to believe him. He could have a recurrence of the disease without having been reexposed.

How can I prevent it?

Condoms, condoms, condoms! Although not 100 percent effective, condoms offer much better protection than using nothing at all. Limit your sexual partners. Do not be embarrassed to look at your partner's genitalia, and if you notice any bumps or lesions, ask him to be examined by a urologist. Remember, teamwork is the only way to conquer this disease.

CHAPTER 9

Gonorrhea: Easy to Treat but Serious if Untreated

More women than you'd think become infected

Key words:

Clap, GC, Drip, Pelvic Inflammatory Disease, Salpingitis, Endometritis

Risks and/or consequences:

- Pelvic inflammatory disease (PID)
- Ectopic pregnancy
- Bartholin gland abscess
- Infertility
- Hysterectomy
- Arthritis

Ten days after having had sexual intercourse, Sharon noticed a slight vaginal discharge. As days went by, her mild abdominal discomfort turned into unbearable pain. Sharon's mother took her to a general practitioner, who upon examination recommended immediate hospitalization. Sharon was given intravenous antibiotics and pain killers, all the while being submitted to a multitude of X-rays and laboratory tests. Her hospitalization lasted four days, and she was released feeling much better and able to resume her normal activities. Her relationship with her boyfriend continued, and although she would experience occasional pain, Sharon never associated this with her previous illness.

Months passed and her pain became severe; Sharon was again admitted into the hospital. Her improvement in the hospital was much slower than the first time, so her doctor called in a gynecologist for a second opinion. At the suggestion of the gynecologist, Sharon underwent an operation known as a laparoscopy. The laparoscopy revealed extensive damage to her reproductive organs: both fallopian tubes were badly scarred rendering her infertile. The gynecologist explained to Sharon that she had pelvic inflammatory disease, and although she had been previously treated, her partner had not. Sharon's partner had unknowingly reinfected her with gonorrhea. Allowing the infection to remain in her body for such a long period of time had produced the scarring.

Sharon's partner was treated but, unfortunately for her, it was too late to preserve her fertility.

What is it?

Gonorrhea is a sexually transmitted disease produced by a bacteria called *Neisseria gonorrhoeae*. Gonorrhea is so widespread that a new infection occurs every twelve seconds. The number of gonorrhea cases has nearly doubled since 1965, with present estimates of 1.3 million new cases reported each year. It is also estimated that another one million new cases go unreported each year. Thirty-five to 45 percent of all PID cases are caused by a gonorrheal infection. Gonorrhea results in the hospitalization of 200,000 women and an estimated yearly cost of $2 billion.

How can I get it?

Gonorrhea is a highly contagious disease requiring minimal sexual contact for transmission. It is transmitted through sexual contact, either through oral or genital sex. Any contact with infected moist tissues such as the vagina, throat, rectum, or urethra can lead to transmission. Vaginal intercourse is the most common way women become infected.

What are the symptoms in women?

Unfortunately, the initial symptoms in a woman may be so vague that up to 80 percent of these women will not recognize their importance. Usually, a week to ten days after infection, she may notice a creamy white discharge produced by the infected cervix. This discharge, although annoying, may not cause any other discomfort beyond burning with urination and frequent urination.

If gonorrhea infects the Bartholin glands at the opening of the vagina, these become swollen and full of pus (abscess). This condition is known as Bartholin gland abscess and is so painful that the patient may be unable to walk or sit.

If untreated, the infection travels into the pelvic area, the uterus, fallopian tubes, and the ovaries. This produces severe abdominal pain, fever, and swollen glands in the groin, or pelvic inflammatory disease. Left untreated this condition can develop into pus pockets, which—unless surgically drained—are fatal.

If a woman develops oral gonorrhea, the symptoms will include a sore throat and a pus-like secretion from her mouth. If she develops a rectal infection, she may experience diarrhea, pus in the stool, and painful bowel movements.

In rare instances, gonorrhea can affect the joints causing an arthritis-like illness with soreness and swelling of the joints.

What are the symptoms in men?

Seven to ten days after exposure to gonorrhea, a man will experience pain when urinating and will also notice a yellowish white penile discharge. Occasionally gonorrhea can spread to the scrotum and prostate, causing excruciating pain. In the case of rectal infection, symptoms including painful bowel movements or diarrhea will develop. Oral infections produce symptoms of irritation and sore throat.

What are the dangers if I get it?

Any gynecologist can recognize a patient with a Bartholin gland abscess just by the way she walks. The pain is so unbearable that she demands immediate attention. The tremendous relief she experiences as soon as the abscess is drained makes the patient thankful to be in the gynecologist's office—something you and I know is rare! There are times when the abscess recurs on its own, necessitating surgical procedures such as marsupialization (deep cleansing).

When gonorrhea causes PID, the consequences can be devastating. When the fallopian tubes become blocked or scarred, fertility is jeopardized. It is estimated that one-fifth of all the women who develop PID will become infertile at that time. Some women with PID will develop a pelvic abscess that can be life-threatening. Abscesses are a major cause of hysterectomies performed on patients with PID. Ectopic pregnancy is another major complication resulting from PID. This can become a serious medical emergency and, if left untreated, will cause death as a result of shock and massive internal bleeding.

A rare consequence of gonorrhea is a hepatitis-like infection called Fitzhugh-Curtis syndrome. This occurs when the infection settles in the liver, causing hepatitis or inflammation.

Chronic pelvic pain caused by scarring may be so severe that the patient must undergo surgical procedures (such as laparoscopies and hysterectomies) to alleviate the pain. I have seen many patients who, even after hysterectomies, continue to experience discomfort.

In men, gonorrhea, if left untreated, may cause scarring and abnormalities of the urethra, causing difficulty urinating.

Women with gonorrhea are significantly more likely than uninfected women to have premature rupture of the amniotic membranes (breaking of the water) and to deliver prematurely. If the baby is delivered through an infected vaginal canal, eye infections in the infant are possible.

How does my doctor find out if I have it?

The doctor may suspect gonorrhea if, upon visual inspection, the cervix appears red and swollen. The vaginal and cervical secretions will alert him to the possibility of the infection. If the patient presents with a Bartholin gland abscess or PID, the doctor should suspect gonorrhea. During the pelvic exam the patient may be extremely tender, also a sign of infection.

If gonorrhea is suspected, the doctor will examine a sample of the cervical or vaginal discharge under the microscope. Sometimes the bacteria will show up immediately, allowing for prompt diagnosis. The doctor will also perform a gonorrheal culture, which involves retrieving a sample of the discharge with a cotton swab and placing it on culture media. The media is sent to a laboratory, and the results are back within forty-eight hours. This test is painless, quick, accurate, and inexpensive. The culture costs $25 or less.

How is it treated?

Antibiotics easily cure this disease. The method of administering the antibiotics varies with the severity of infection. Most often two shots of penicillin are required, or antibiotics such as doxycycline or ampicillin may be used for seven to ten days. This regimen is used to treat uncomplicated cases of gonorrhea. When PID is present, hospitalization with intravenous antibiotics is required. Partners must be treated accordingly in order to achieve a complete cure.

How can I prevent it?

Condoms are an effective method of preventing gonorrhea. Barrier contraceptives like the diaphragm may prevent the spread of the disease; spermicides used along with these barrier methods have shown great promise in reducing the chances of gonoccocal infection. Limit your number of sexual partners and learn to recognize symptoms in your partner.

CHAPTER 10

Genital Herpes:
One in Six Adults Has It

Managed properly, it need
not ruin lives or relationships

Key words:

Blisters, Cold Sores, Genital Herpes, HSV

Risks and/or consequences:

- Cervical cancer
- Cesarean section
- Blindness

Pamela thought she was developing a yeast infection. Her vaginal area was swollen and red. She made an appointment with her gynecologist for the next day. By the time the doctor examined Pamela, her vulva had five painful blisters. The diagnosis was simple: herpes. Her initial response was shame and frustration at having contracted a disease which carries so much stigma and for which there is no cure. How could she tell future partners she was infected with the herpes virus? What were the implications for childbearing? Pamela had many questions and fears. With the guidance of her doctor and many support groups, she learned that the disease can be controlled and that most patients lead a perfectly normal life.

What is it?

Herpes is a common term for an infection caused by the herpes simplex virus (HSV).

There are two types of herpes simplex virus. Type 1 (HSV 1) generally causes cold sores or fever blisters; Type 2 (HSV 2) causes genital herpes. There is evidence that some genital herpes may be caused by the HSV 1 virus and that some oral herpes may be caused by HSV 2 when sexual partners engage in oral-genital relations. The Centers for Disease Control estimates that there are 500,000 new cases of genital herpes in the United States each year. Genital herpes is epidemic in this country. Thirty million people are estimated to have genital herpes, which translates to one out of every six adults. Herpes-related physicians' office visits have increased ten-fold over the last fifteen years. After the initial outbreak, herpes can recur up to four times a year. These recurrences are usually triggered by illness, fatigue, stress, menstruation, or sexual intercourse. Studies show that for many individuals, these recurrences decrease as time goes by.

How can I get it?

The disease is transmitted by coming into contact with another person who has herpes lesions. This is almost always through sexual contact. In general, if there are no visible lesions, the person is not contagious. However, a small percentage of the time, men and women with genital herpes may be contagious even though they do not show any signs or symptoms of the disease. Thus, it is possible for them to infect their partners without having active blisters.

If a person has a cold sore and puts their mouth on their partner's genitals, it is possible for their partner to develop genital herpes. Likewise, cold sores may develop after engaging in oral-genital sex with an infected partner.

It is theoretically possible for a woman to be infected from secretions on a toilet seat. However, in order for this extremely uncommon situation to occur, the secretions on the toilet seat must still be warm and moist and come in contact with broken skin. Rules of hygiene and common sense make this an unlikely scenario.

What are the symptoms in women?

The initial infection of herpes occurs within three weeks after sexual contact with a contagious person. During the first outbreak, the infected area becomes extremely painful and swollen. An itchy sensation begins in the vulva or vagina and is accompanied by fever, headaches, or a flu-like illness. The blisters that follow look like clear, raised bumps and are filled with a fluid that is highly contagious. These blisters or sores can last from one week to ten days. Thereafter, they rupture and heal as new skin tissue forms. After this occurs, the virus becomes dormant within the nervous system. The immune system develops weapons against the virus that make subsequent outbreaks less severe. There are usually fewer sores (which heal faster), and the flu-like symptoms of the first outbreak are seldom present.

What are the symptoms in men?

In males, pain, tenderness or an itching sensation precede the blisters that localize on the penis. The blisters may also form on the thighs or buttocks. Other symptoms are the same in men as in women.

What are the dangers if I get it?

Genital herpes is an inconvenient and uncomfortable disease that fortunately causes very few medical complications. Most of the damage that herpes does to a woman comes from the unwarranted social stigma associated with the disease. Herpes directly attacks a woman's sense of control over her body. The disease comes and goes at will, giving the patient a sense of helplessness.

Studies show a very slight increase in the risk of developing cervical cancer due to the virus. We now know that, although the risk does exist, its importance has been greatly exaggerated.

If the virus comes in contact with the eye (by touching the eye after touching an active lesion), it can cause herpes keratitis, a form of herpes that can cause blindness if left untreated. Such infections are rare; using common sense and good hygiene will prevent them. Aside from occasional eye complications and the emotional reaction, medical implications for men are virtually nonexistent.

Very rarely, pregnant women who have active lesions present in the birth canal at the time of delivery transmit the disease to their baby. When this happens, the baby may suffer damage to the brain and central nervous system. A high percentage of herpes-infected babies will die within the first year of life. The harmful effects to the infant may be avoided by an elective cesarean section at the time of delivery.

How does my doctor find out if I have it?

An experienced gynecologist should be able to diagnose a herpes outbreak by the history a patient gives and by looking at the herpes blister. Laboratory tests may be used to confirm the diagnosis. If a culture taken from the secretions of a blister proves positive, the patient has herpes. If it is negative, the patient may or may not have the disease, since the culture can be wrong up to 20 percent of the time. The culture is painless; the results take up to seven days to come back from the laboratory. Genital herpes may also be diagnosed by microscopic examination of a scraping from a blister. Blood tests are not useful in determining whether you have contracted herpes and presently are not recommended for the diagnosis of the disease.

How is it treated?

There is no known cure for genital herpes. During an outbreak of herpes, the patient must keep the lesions as clean and as dry as possible. Analgesics such as aspirin may be used to control the discomfort. The only medicine available is called Zovirax (acyclovir) and may be used in capsule or ointment form. It does not cure the disease but in most patients provides substantial relief by shortening the duration of the outbreak. For recurrent outbreaks of herpes, Zovirax capsules can greatly reduce the number of outbreaks; in many cases, Zovirax completely prevents them if the patient takes the medication daily as prescribed by her doctor.

How can I prevent it?

Never have sex with a partner who has obvious herpes blisters. If you are not sure that you or your partner is free of infection, use latex condoms along with spermicidal foams and jellies containing nonoxynol-9. These help prevent transmission and may also kill the herpes simplex virus.

CHAPTER 11

Syphilis: Deadly if Untreated

Early detection is the key to cure

Key words:

Chancre (pronounced "shanker"), Spirochete

Risks and/or consequences:

- Blindness
- Paralysis
- Senility or dementia
- Loss of feeling in legs
- Central nervous system disease
- Death

Thinking that syphilis was rare gave me a false sense of security as an intern. It was with total shock and disbelief that I once watched a baby die: I will never forget his grotesque features and the quickness of his death. His mother had not had proper maternal care—perhaps out of ignorance, perhaps because she could not afford it. To think that this baby would have been born healthy if his mother had received just one injection of penicillin still saddens me.

What is it?

Syphilis is a sexually transmitted disease caused by *Treponema pallidum,* a spirochete (or spiral-shaped bacterium). Syphilis has been around for centuries creating health nightmares for most of the world. It was not until the 1940s, when penicillin became widely used, that this disease was finally contained. Syphilis was largely forgotten until the 1980s, when poverty, drug abuse, and the decline in health care in inner cities created an upwardly spiraling trend. Reported incidents of syphilis have doubled since 1984, ranging between 130,000 to 150,000 new cases each year.

How can I get it?

Syphilis is transmitted from open sores or rashes during sexual activity, including sexual intercourse, and oral and anal sex. The bacteria easily penetrate the walls of the vagina, the linings of the mouth and rectum, and—in rare occurrences—the skin itself.

What are the symptoms in women?

Syphilis develops in three stages that can last a lifetime if untreated. The most common and noticeable symptom of the first stage of the disease is a painless sore called a chancre that usually appears three to four weeks after contact. The chancre is red, firm, and rises above the skin. If the sore is inside the vagina, it is more difficult to detect. The chancre heals four to six weeks after appearing, leaving a thin scar in the area. This scar is extremely hard to see. The second stage begins about six to twelve weeks after infection; the patient experiences a flu-like illness with symptoms ranging from fever to a loss of appetite. Many of these patients develop skin conditions that include spots on the palms and soles, small red bumps, and gray plaques in the mucous membranes of the mouth, vulva, and vagina. These growths may become ulcerated and may ooze fluid. They are extremely infectious. Secondary syphilis may last for about one year and will pass even without treatment. At this time the signs of syphilis will disappear spontaneously and the third (latent) stage begins, lasting from two years to a lifetime. It is during this third, noncontagious stage that syphilis produces devastating medical problems in almost every part of the body. It may cause paralysis, senility, loss of equilibrium, blindness, and loss of feeling in the legs.

What are the symptoms in men?

Men experience the same symptoms as women, the main difference being that the initial chancre will most likely appear on the penis, enabling the patient to recognize the disease sooner. Syphilis is one of the few nonsexist sexually transmitted diseases: it is equally devastating to men and women.

What are the dangers if I get it?

During the first two stages of syphilis, the dangers to you and your partner are not serious. It is during the third stage of the disease that it does its greatest damage. Once incurred, organ damage sometimes cannot be reversed even with treatment, meaning that the paralysis, dementia, and blindness are permanent. Left untreated, this disease eventually kills most of its victims.

The unborn child of a syphilitic mother is affected during all three stages of syphilis. Babies can develop syphilis while still in utero. Such pregnancies often end in miscarriages or stillbirths. Other infected babies die soon after birth. Those who survive are often born with multiple abnormalities such as an enlarged liver, spleen, eye or ear damage, as well as many cosmetic deformities.

How does my doctor find out if I have it?

Primary syphilis may be readily diagnosed by the microscopic examination of the spirochete in the chancre. This is a simple and inexpensive test. The most reliable method of diagnosis is a blood test, which takes about two days to come back from the lab and costs about $15 to $25. This test is highly accurate but may take as long as six months after initial sexual contact to register a positive finding. It is advisable for a patient who suspects exposure to syphilis, to repeat the test after six months to ensure that she is infection-free.

How is it treated?

Penicillin is the most effective mode of treatment. A single injection will cure the patient during the first and second stages of the disease. In stage three, the treatment includes antibiotics and other forms of therapy to alleviate the symptoms and damage that the disease has already done. When the disease has affected the central nervous system, syphilis is usually untreatable. Successful treatment of syphilis does not prevent reinfection.

How can I prevent it?

Using a condom during intercourse reduces the risk of contracting syphilis. Abstinence, as well as limiting the number of sexual partners, will also diminish the risk. Remember that any lesion—whether a bump or painless sore—is not a normal occurrence in a man. When in doubt, seek medical help for yourself and your partner.

CHAPTER 12

Hepatitis B: It's Spreading and Can Be Dangerous

The only STD for which we have a vaccine

Key words:

Serum Hepatitis, Liver Infection

Risks and/or consequences:

- Liver cancer
- Chronic hepatitis
- Cirrhosis or liver damage

Michelle thought she had the flu and stayed in bed for four days. In spite of all this rest, she felt more tired than before; and now she noticed that the whites of her eyes were beginning to turn yellow. On the advice of her roommate, she went to her college infirmary, where she was given a blood test that diagnosed her with hepatitis B. The physician suggested her boyfriend also be tested. Much to their surprise, he was identified as a carrier of the disease. He looked and felt healthy but never realized he was infected with hepatitis B. Michelle was lucky: the infection did not do any long-term damage, but due to the lengthy ill-ness, she was forced to miss a semester of her college work.

What is it?

Hepatitis B is an infection of the liver caused by the hepatitis B virus (HBV). Hepatitis B isn't generally thought of as a sexually transmitted disease, but it should be. The virus infects an estimated 350,000 people in the United States each year and kills 6,000. Sex is the leading mode of transmission.

In previous years, those affected most by hepatitis B were homosexuals but—apparently in response to AIDS-inspired precautions—their rate of infection has dramatically decreased. Heterosexual transmission, on the other hand, has surged by 43 percent over the last ten years.

How can I get it?

Hepatitis B is most commonly transmitted through sexual intercourse. This occurs by contact with the sperm of an infected male or the menstrual blood of an infected female. Nonsexual transmission occurs through blood transfusions, contaminated IV needles, or contact with saliva.

What are the symptoms?

Common symptoms of hepatitis B include weakness, loss of appetite, nausea, dark urine, fever, jaundice (yellowing of the skin), and abdominal discomfort. Some patients describe the symptoms as "the worst flu I've ever had." In rare cases persons infected with HBV will develop no symptoms. Such persons become carriers of the disease and are able to transmit the virus to others without knowing it.

What are the dangers if I get it?

Although most people recover naturally from this disease without any lasting effects, hepatitis B is potentially dangerous. An estimated 10 percent of HBV-infected people develop chronic liver disease, which involves progressive liver failure and eventual death. A small percentage of these chronic hepatitis B patients will develop liver cancer. The majority of these patients die within five years.

A pregnant woman may pass the virus on to a newborn during delivery. These infants may become chronic hepatitis B carriers, with a higher incidence of liver disease.

How does my doctor find out if I have it?

Hepatitis B is diagnosed by a blood test that can be performed in your physician's office. The results are quick, and the cost of the test ranges from $15 to $25.

How is it treated?

There is no cure for hepatitis B. The treatment consists of supportive measures such as rest and a high-calorie diet. Recently, antiviral drugs such as interferon have been used to slow the progress of the disease. The results of such treatment have been mixed. However, once a patient has contracted hepatitis B, she eventually develops an immunity to the disease and cannot be reinfected.

How can I prevent it?

Hepatitis B is the only sexually transmitted disease for which we have a vaccine. In years to come you will see a tremendous educational push to inform the public about the dangers of hepatitis B and the availability of this proven vaccine. The vaccine must be taken in three visits spread over six months. It is easily attainable in doctors' offices, health clinics, and college infirmaries.

The use of a condom during sexual intercourse reduces the risk of contracting or transmitting hepatitis B sexually. The risk of contracting hepatitis B nonsexually can be reduced by avoiding contact with the body fluids of an infected person, by not sharing IV drug needles, and in general by using the same precautions used to reduce the risk of contracting HIV.

CHAPTER 13

Vaginitis: Gardnerella, Trichomoniasis, Yeast Infections

Facts that can prevent many visits to your doctor

Key words:
Trich, Yeast, Bacterial, Clue Cells, Candidiasis, Moniliasis

Risks and/or consequences:
- Itching
- Vaginal discharge
- Vaginal pain
- Abnormal Pap smear

Not a single week goes by in my practice in which I do not encounter a new patient who states, "My vaginal infection keeps coming back—my previous doctor told me I was susceptible to them." Unless those patients are severely diabetic or take daily antibiotics, they have been given the wrong information. When properly diagnosed and treated, vaginitis should be an infrequent reason for you to visit your gynecologist.

What is it?

Vaginitis is a term used to refer to various infections of the vagina. For the purpose of this discussion, I will limit my discussion to the three most common types of vaginitis: Trichomoniasis, Gardnerella, and Candida.

Trichomonas vaginalis is a sexually transmitted parasite present in the vagina and the male urethra.

Gardnerella vaginalis is almost invariably transmitted sexually. It may be present in the vagina and male urethra.

The fungus *Candida albicans* causes candidiasis (also called moniliasis) or yeast. Candidiasis is not a sexually transmitted disease in the true sense of the word, but many patients suffer reinfection if their partner is not treated.

It is estimated that as many as 40 percent of all females will be infected with some type of vaginitis during their lifetimes. Vaginitis accounts for more physician visits than any other sexually transmitted disorder. In 1988 the Centers for Disease Control reported about eleven million office visits for vaginitis. (I know this is a conservative estimate since physicians do not report these diseases.)

How can I get it?

When the cause of a vaginitis is sexual transmission, such as trichomonas or gardnerella, infection occurs by direct sexual contract. A yeast infection usually occurs when there is an overgrowth of the yeast in the vagina. This can be caused by the use of antibiotics (which decrease vaginal bacteria, which otherwise keeps yeast in control). Many other factors can increase your risk for a yeast infection: tampons, birth control pills, douching, bath oils, and frequent tub baths. Although not considered a sexually transmitted disease, yeast infections can be transmitted from one partner to another during sexual intercourse.

What are the symptoms in women?

In general the symptoms of vaginitis—regardless of the source of the infection—are similar. These include itching, burning, pain during intercourse, vaginal odor, and vaginal discharge. Trichomoniasis is characterized by a watery, frothy vaginal discharge. Itching is intense. Gardnerella causes a white or grayish discharge accompanied by a pungent, fishy smell. Yeast infections do not smell but produce a cottage cheese-like discharge, which causes extreme itching and irritation.

What are the symptoms in men?

Men usually have no symptoms, but when they occur they may include burning with urination, and penile discharge. Yeast infections can cause a rash on the penis.

What are the dangers if I get it?

The medical consequences of these infections include abnormal pap smears, chronic vaginal irritation, and pain during intercourse. For most patients the consequences are emotional and/or financial rather than medical. They are frustrated by the discomfort, as well as by the multiple office visits and their associated costs.

How does my doctor find out if I have it?

Vaginitis is easily diagnosed by microscopic examination of the discharge. This is called a "wet mount" and is performed in a doctor's office. The results are immediate, and the cost is usually minimal ($5 to $10). Many gynecologists do not even charge for this test.

How is it treated?

Treatment for trichomoniasis usually involves oral medication such as Flagyl. Gardnerella is treated with antibiotics or vaginal creams. Yeast infection treatments include vaginal creams and/or vaginal suppositories, many of which are nonprescription (Monistat 7 and Gyne-Lotrimin). Unless you are 100 percent sure you have a yeast infection, do not self-medicate with these vaginal creams. If both partners are treated appropriately, relapses are uncommon. Never accept a prescription treatment for a vaginal infection without inquiring if your partner also needs to be treated.

How can I prevent it?

The chances of contracting nonsexually transmitted forms of vaginitis are minimized by careful genital hygiene and the avoidance of vaginal irritants. Do not use feminine hygiene sprays or powders. Douching is not—and should not be— a part of feminine hygiene. Limit tub baths, the use of nylon underpants, and foods rich in sugars.

Sexually transmitted forms of vaginitis are most effectively avoided by limiting your chance of reinfection. This is best accomplished by demanding that your partner receives treatment even if he has no symptoms. In short, if you are treated for trichomoniasis or gardnerella without your partner also being treated, you may as well set up another appointment while you're there because you'll be back.

CHAPTER 14

Rare or Less Familiar STDs

Some are serious, some merely annoying

In this chapter I will briefly discuss some uncommon sexually transmitted diseases. They range from being annoying to medically serious and, although rare, still warrant discussion.

Pubic lice (crabs, pediculosis)

Pubic lice inhabit the genital area and are transmitted by close personal contact. They may also be transmitted via the clothing or bed sheets of an infected person. Unlike head lice, pubic lice infect only the hair of the pubis (genital area). Unsanitary personal habits foster the spread of this disease. Although infestation with pubic lice is of no medical danger, the itching can be so severe that the patient will scratch the area raw, which may cause open sores and scabs. These sores can become infected by normal skin bacteria, creating boils or abscesses. Pubic lice can be easily gotten rid of using over-the-counter medicines or prescription lotions (such as Kwell).

Scabies

Scabies is caused by a mite *(Sarcoptes scabiei)*, which is a parasite of the skin. The mite burrows into soft skins of the body, such as skin folds, the penis, or nipples. Scabies is transmitted by close contact, such as sharing a bed or clothing, or sexual contact with an infected person. It causes intense itching usually at night. The resulting scratching may cause open sores that eventually become infected. Treatment involves prescription lotion (Kwell) and careful cleansing of infected clothes and bedding.

Molluscum contagiosum

Molluscum contagiosum is an infectious disease of the skin affecting the face, arms, genitals, abdomen, and thighs. It is caused by a mildly contagious virus transmitted through skin-to-skin contact. Molluscum appears as small bumps resembling pimples; they do not hurt and are not dangerous. The gynecologist will reserve treatment for those patients who exhibit large numbers of bumps. In these cases, molluscum is treated by scraping out the growths.

Chancroid

Chancroid is a bacterial infection of the genitourinary tract in which a rapidly growing ulcerated lesion forms on the genitalia. It is caused by the bacteria *Haemophilus ducreyi* and is usually transmitted through sexual intercourse. The ulcers are extremely painful, affecting the penis and the opening of the vagina. If untreated, chancroid can cause painful and extensive tissue destruction with abscess formation in the groin. Treatment with tetracycline usually achieves a complete cure. In the last decade, the number of reported chancroid cases has doubled and, because the disease may be a facilitator in the transmission of AIDS, increasing attention is being paid to it.

Lymphogranuloma venereum (LGV)

LGV is a sexually transmitted disease caused by *Chlamydia trachomatis,* serotypes 1, 2, 3. It is mainly found in tropical and subtropical climates. LGV causes sores in the genital area that lead to a unilateral abscess in the groin. These abscesses produce scar formations with chronic drainage, which in turn may cause blockage of the lymphatic vessels leading to swelling and ulceration. These complications of LGV may involve the vagina and the rectum. Tetracyclines will cure this disease but may not resolve the rectal scars.

Granuloma inguinale (GI)

GI is a chronic bacterial infection caused by the bacteria *Donovania granulomatis.* It is usually found in tropical and subtropical areas and is transmitted by sexual contact. In the female, painless ulcer-type lesions arise on the vulva and vagina that may gradually encompass the entire pubic area. These lesions may bleed and cause secondary infection, resulting in large amounts of tissue destruction. In the male, these lesions appear on the penis, scrotum, and groin. GI is easily treated with tetracycline.

Mycoplasma homonis and ureaplasma urealyticum infections

These organisms are part of the vaginal flora of most women. They have been implicated in certain cases of spontaneous abortions (miscarriages) and infertility. Their role in pelvic infections has not been established, but I believe they may prove to be far more serious than we give them credit for, accounting for that group of patients with PID for which we have no causative agent. Treatment with tetracycline results in complete cure.

PART FOUR

CHAPTER 15

If You Have an STD: Dealing with Your Doctor and Your Partner

The quality of care you get will depend on the questions you ask

Maria and Robert are an engaged couple with a bright future. I say that because they have already come through a challenge that would strain most marriages, and it has brought them closer together. Here is their story in their own words:

Maria: I had been having a lot of pain in my abdomen, and Robert kept telling me to go to the doctor. But I'm one of those women who learned in childhood to be strong, so even when I am really suffering, I say, "Oh, it's not that bad."

Robert: Although Maria was in pain, she was still working out and even doing sit-ups. I'd say, "We'll go to the doctor next week, right?" She'd say, "Maybe. I'll wait and see whether it goes away on its own." She toughed it out for at least six weeks.

Maria: Finally, when I couldn't even sleep, I made an appointment with a gynecologist. The doctor said I had pelvic inflammatory disease (PID) and that my fertility had probably been damaged. He wanted to determine the extent of the damage by doing a laparoscopy (examination of the pelvic organs by means of a laparoscope, a thin viewing scope, which is inserted through one or more small incisions). He asked me to make another appointment so he could explain everything to me.

Robert: Maria never said, "Please come with me to talk to my gynecologist." When she told me the doctor's diagnosis and that he wanted to operate, I said, "I'm going unless you don't want me to be there." I had a lot of reasons for wanting to come along. Once I went to a doctor for back pain, and he didn't even want to spend five minutes with me. I'll never go back to him because I don't think he gave me the service I paid for. So I asked Maria whether she trusted him, and she said she liked him, but I wanted to check out the doctor for myself and maybe urge her to get a second opinion. I don't know much about female problems, but I would have gone to meet a doctor who wanted to operate on her foot, so why not see *this* doctor?

I also went with Maria to find out about what she had and what care she needed. She would have done the same for me. It's a team effort and we both have to beat this, but I never thought of being there as an obligation or a responsibility. It's just where I had to be. If she needs help, I'm there.

Maria: The doctor took at least an hour to explain everything to us, including the news that PID is sexually transmitted. I had heard that sexually transmitted diseases (STDs) show up right away in guys, but we learned that these STDs can hide for a while, especially in women. Who caught the STD first turned out to be the last thing of importance on our minds. In our situation, we may never know, but we weren't really concerned with blame. We were more worried about the effect of PID on our future plans for a pregnancy.

Robert: Our meeting with the doctor turned out to be educational in itself. At first I didn't know what questions to ask other than "Gee, what's the matter?" and "How can we fix it?" Also, the female reproductive system was pretty hazy in my mind. I'm visually oriented, so I asked the doctor to explain things using pictures. That way I could visualize Maria's problem and what the doctor was proposing. His explanations helped a lot in easing some fears I had and brought out others I had never thought about.

If I hadn't learned about the laparoscopy Maria was about to undergo, I could have assumed that the situation was a lot less critical than it was. Also, if I hadn't gotten involved, Maria might have hidden her fears from me. Especially if she didn't seem too shaken up, I might not have offered her much support. But because I was a part of all the discussions, I didn't think of the surgery as merely Maria's problem. We were facing surgery together as a couple.

Maria: It's a good thing Robert came along to that second appointment, because he thought of questions to ask, and he heard things that I missed. The possibility that I might have lost some of my fertility really threw me at first. I think if he had not been there, I would have come home and announced, "The doctor says I can't have any children." Instead, Robert was able to remind me that although the doctor said I probably won't be able to have babies without help, there are several options we can try when we are ready.

Robert: When we brought up the question of Maria's possibly getting a second opinion, her gynecologist said that if we felt we needed one, to go ahead. That's worth something to me. Getting bids is a common business practice, so why shouldn't patients do something similar and consult more than one doctor before having surgery?

Maria: The morning I went in for the laparoscopy, I was really scared. But the doctor's explanations helped a lot because I knew there would be only two minor incisions. As expected, he found I had scars everywhere in my pelvis that were clogging the fallopian tubes. Robert cried when the doctor first told him about the damage PID had caused. But he has never said anything about his taking on the responsibility for a disease I might have contracted before I ever met him.

Robert: I went along for Maria's postoperative checkup. I didn't do that just in a spirit of "I'm going to help you through this." I went with her because I needed to find out how things were going and if there were any problems. The doctor says that if we want to have children, she will need more surgery from an infertility expert, or we could get into an in vitro program. But as long as Maria doesn't suffer the pain she had, it doesn't matter to me whether we can or cannot have children naturally. We can adopt. We can do other things.

Maybe you are reading this chapter because you noticed symptoms that could have been caused by an STD, and you went straight to a gynecologist. Now the tests have all been run and there is no doubt: you have an STD. What do you do now?

Now more than ever, you need straight talk—between you and your gynecologist, and between you and your partner. You need to allow yourself to have whatever feelings come up and to express them. Also, you must educate yourself about the disease.

If you have already created a partnership with a competent gynecologist, you should have a strong source of support to help you through the process that lies ahead. Even if you don't have a doctor-patient partnership yet, your gynecologist can provide the care you deserve, as long as you handle your share of the responsibility for making that happen.

This chapter is intended to help you in the area in which you may need the most help. Your main responsibility right now is to ask a lot of questions. From experience, I can say that if you just found out that you have an STD, you probably aren't in the best position to come up with all the questions you need to ask. You probably don't have enough information to ask all the right questions. What's more, you probably won't remember all you need to ask while you are still at your doctor's office.

The following list of questions can be a guideline in your talks with your doctor. You will probably want to list additional questions that relate to your own situation. Remember, it is your responsibility to ask these questions and your right to have them answered.

Questions regarding my condition

What specifically do I have?
- What's its name?

Is it serious?
- What are the risks and consequences of having this?
- What damage has already been done?
- Will it affect my ability to get pregnant?

How long could I have had it?

Might I have other STDs?

Can I pass this disease on to someone else?

Do I need to avoid sex while I'm being treated?

Can I be cured of this disease? If so:
- What are the treatment options (medication, surgery)?

  If surgical or invasive procedures are recommended, see Chapter 16.

- What risks are involved in the treatment?
- What is the prognosis (likely outcome) with treatment?
- How long will it take to know I am cured?
- What are the risks and possible side effects?
- How much will the treatment cost?
- What kind of follow-up care will I need?

Once I am cured, can I catch the disease again?
- If so, how can I prevent that?
- Is there any medication or treatment to prevent recurrences?

If this disease can't be cured, can treatment relieve the symptoms?

Do you have any written information about this STD?

Questions regarding my partner

What should I tell my partner about getting tested and treated?

Will you explain the disease and treatment to him and/or refer him to a physician?

What are the risks and consequences of his having this STD?

What questions should he ask his doctor?

Will you talk to his doctor?

After he is treated, what precautions will we need to take?

Hopefully, a simple course of antibiotics will have solved your problem. But for those times when further testing and/or treatment is needed, the following chapter will give you an overview of various procedures your doctor may suggest.

CHAPTER 16

Surgery for Diagnosis or Treatment of an STD

Everything you need to find out—before and after

Recently a panel of nurses let down their hair and shared some straight talk of their own on what patients facing gynecological surgery need to know. Here are some of their comments:

> I had a patient who said to me, "I don't know why my doctor admitted me. I don't feel that bad." When I questioned her, she knew absolutely nothing about why she was scheduled for surgery other than that she was having pain. I said, "I suggest that you ask him why he put you in here." But she said she didn't feel comfortable asking him any questions.

> I can't tell you how many times I've had a patient come in for surgery, and when I asked her what procedures she was having done, she couldn't begin to tell me. I'll see that she's signed a consent form to have certain organs removed, and she'll say, "Oh! I didn't think he was going to take my tubes and ovaries out."

It's so frustrating when a patient asks me basic questions about what her problem is and what her doctor is going to do during surgery. As a nurse, I'm not allowed to tell her anything. All I can do is suggest that she write down her questions and take them up with her physician.

I always ask a surgical patient, "Do you understand what you're going to have done today?" When she says yes, I ask her to tell me, because I want to hear that she knows what's on the consent form she signed. The conversation will go like this: "He's going to take out my uterus." "How is he going to do it?" "I think he's going to make an incision." You have to walk patients through it to make sure they really do know. Some patients really don't understand what is going to happen, and I've had to call the physician and tell him that he needs to come and talk to his patient. It's not my place or my responsibility to discuss her surgery.

When a patient wakes up in the recovery room, usually the first question she asks is, "What did the doctor find?" That's such a hard question for a nurse to be asked, because we aren't allowed to say anything. We know that she's going to keep asking questions every time we go in her room, and all we can say is, "Wait until your doctor gets here." The problem is, sometimes the doctor doesn't visit her until the next morning. I feel bad when I know a patient is going to have to wait all night with her questions.

You can tell when a doctor has done a good job of educating the patient preoperatively. His patients are better informed, they know what to expect, and as a result, they recover much better.

No surgical procedure is minor when you are the one who is going to be on the operating table. For many patients facing surgery, two of their greatest anxieties are that they'll be in an environment that is intimidating because it is so unfamiliar, and that they'll be in a situation they find terrifying because they have to relinquish control over their bodies to strangers wearing masks and white coats.

Because you are a patient who has learned to be in partnership with her doctor, your surgery can be an entirely different experience. No matter whether you undergo a procedure in your gynecologist's office or in the hospital, no matter whether you have same-day surgery or stay overnight in the hospital, no matter whether you receive a local or general anesthetic, the more you know about what is going to happen before, during, and after surgery, the better the care you will receive and the quicker you will recover.

Regardless of who handles your surgical procedure— your gynecologist in his office or a team of hospital physicians and nurses—you have the right to a thorough briefing every step of the way. As you exercise that right, you have the same responsibilities I have been reiterating throughout this book: to ask a lot of questions and to make sure that they get answered. This chapter will guide you through that process.

The rest of this chapter is divided into two parts. First, I'll suggest the most important questions to ask at every stage of your experience as a surgical patient. Second, I will provide some background information on the procedures your gynecologist is most likely to recommend if you have had an abnormal Pap smear or need treatment for an STD.

Questions to ask if your doctor recommends surgery

A relative of mine recently underwent a surgical procedure called a laparotomy to remove an ovarian cyst. Although her gynecologist is well respected, he doesn't feel comfortable doing some of the latest procedures. He should have recommended a less drastic procedure known as a laparoscopy and referred my relative to another physician, but his ego got in the way. My relative did get a second opinion, and the doctor she consulted recommended a laparoscopy, but because she was too hesitant to hurt her own doctor's feelings, she went ahead and had the surgery he recommended. Here is the difference between the operation she had and the operation she should have had:

Laparotomy	Laparoscopy
open abdominal surgery	abdomen not opened
one large incision; a long scar	two small incisions; negligible scars
three- to four-day hospital stay	same-day, or outpatient, surgery
pain of major surgery	minor pain
great chance of infection	chance of infection minor
long recovery period	quick return to normal activities
more expensive	less expensive

As you can see, these surgeries are very different. I know most of you would have chosen a laparoscopy if you had been presented with both choices and the pros and cons of each. If you are faced with the prospect of an operation, you should educate yourself on the ways a problem can be treated surgically and allow your physician to help you make an intelligent decision. It is vital to understand that some physicians don't keep up with the latest technology and may not necessarily tell you that they feel uncomfortable performing a newer procedure. A good physician will explain all the surgical options available, whether he knows how to perform them or not.

Figure 3 on the next page is an example of a typical opera-tive permit (also called a surgical consent form) for a total abdominal hysterectomy. Look how complicated this form is! All operations have a similar operative permit that you must sign, with the same unfamiliar medical terminology.

Imagine that your doctor recommends surgery, and you agree without any discussion because "the doctor knows best." Right before they wheel you down to the operating room, someone waves this form under your nose and asks for your signature. You scan it and see, for the first time, the risks and hazards associated with the surgery you are about to have, as well as the risks associated with the anesthetic. Can you honestly say you wouldn't hesitate before signing this form?

My point is that you cannot make an informed choice to have an operation if you wait until right before the surgery to discuss its risks and hazards. The only acceptable time and place to discuss all the pros and cons of surgery is in your gynecologist's office *before* you make your choice. Remember, in gynecology the vast majority of surgical pro-cedures are not emergency operations. In most cases you will be able to exercise your right to take as much time as you need to ask questions and weigh all the alternatives before making an informed decision.

Almost every day, new gynecological procedures are developed. Is your doctor keeping up? Obviously, he won't recommend procedures he doesn't yet know how to do. Give yourself time to read up on the procedures that are being done for your problem. If, as in the case of my rela-tive, you need a cyst or an ovary removed, can your doctor take it out through the little incision involved in a lapa-roscopy instead of putting you through major surgery in a hospital? Look around for a second—and even a third—opinion. Consult physicians from different age groups. After all, a very young doctor might be too keen to do the latest

DISCLOSURE AND CONSENT
MEDICAL AND SURGICAL PROCEDURES

TO THE PATIENT: *You have the right, as a patient, to be informed about your condition and the recommended surgical, medical, or diagnostic procedure to be used so that you may make the decision whether or not to undergo the procedure after knowing the risks and hazards involved. This disclosure is not meant to scare or alarm you; it is simply an effort to make you better informed so you may give or withhold your consent to the procedure.*

I (we) voluntarily request Dr. _____
as my physician, and such associates, technical assistants and other health care providers as they may deem necessary, to treat my condition which has been explained to me as: _____

I (we) understand that the following surgical, medical, and/or diagnostic procedures are planned for me and I (we) voluntarily consent and authorize these procedures: _Abdominal hysterectomy (total)._

I (we) understand that my physician may discover other or different conditions which require additional or different procedures than those planned. I (we) authorize my physician, and such associates, technical assistants and other health care providers to perform such other procedures which are advisable in their professional judgment.

I (we) (do) (do not) consent to the use of blood and blood products as deemed necessary.

I (we) understand that no warranty or guarantee has been made to me as to result or cure.

Just as there may be risks and hazards in continuing my present condition without treatment, there are also risks and hazards related to the performance of the surgical, medical, and/or diagnostic procedures planned for me. I (we) realize that common to surgical, medical, and/or diagnostic procedures is the potential for infection, blood clots in veins and lungs, hemorrhage, allergic reactions, and even death. I (we) also realize that the following risks and hazards may occur in connection with this particular procedure:
1. Uncontrollable leakage of urine.
2. Injury to bladder.
3. Sterility.
4. Injury to the tube between the kidney and the bladder.
5. Injury to the bowel and/or intestinal obstruction.

I (we) understand that anesthesia involves additional risks and hazards but I (we) request the use of anesthetics for the relief and protection from pain during the planned and additional procedures. I (we) realize the anesthesia may have to be changed possibly without explanation to me (us).

I (we) understand that certain complications may result from the use of any anesthetic including respiratory problems, drug reaction, paralysis, brain damage or even death. Other risks and hazards which may result from the use of general anesthetics range from minor discomfort to injury to vocal cords, teeth or eyes. I (we) understand that other risks and hazards resulting from spinal or epidural anesthetics include headache and chronic pain.

I (we) have been given an opportunity to ask questions about my condition, alternative forms of anesthesia and treatment, risks of nontreatment, the procedures to be used, and the risks and hazards involved, and I (we) believe that I (we) have sufficient information to give this informed consent.

I (we) certify this form has been fully explained to me, that I (we) have read it or have had it read to me, that the blank spaces have been filled in, and that I (we) understand its contents.

DATE: _____ TIME: _____ A.M. / P.M.

PATIENT/OTHER LEGALLY RESPONSIBLE PERSON SIGN

WITNESS:

Name

Address (Street or P.O. Box)

City, State, Zip Code

Figure 3

procedures, while a doctor who's been in practice for a long time might not be current on recent advances in the field.

Although gynecologists do countless biopsies and other procedures during their careers, you may have just one procedure in a lifetime. We won't judge you for asking questions. The following is a guide to the initial questions you should ask if your doctor recommends surgery.

Why do I need this procedure? What is it going to accomplish?

Please describe what you will do during surgery.

Are there any other treatment options?

What are the risks?
- Can we go over the surgical consent form before the day of the surgery?

How many times have you done this procedure?

Will this procedure be done as outpatient surgery, or will I need to be hospitalized?
- If the latter is true, how long will I be in the hospital?

How long is the usual recovery period?

What kind of follow-up care will I need?

How much pain can I expect after surgery?

What will postoperative pain management involve?

Will anyone be assisting you in the surgery?
- If any doctors-in-training will assist, what part of the surgery will they do? (You have the right to refuse to have doctors-in-training assisting in your surgery.)

Will you visit me after the surgery? If so, how frequently?

When can the surgery be scheduled?

What will the procedure cost? What charges will that include?
   (The anesthesiologist will bill separately, and so will any surgical assistants.)

What is involved in filing an insurance claim for this procedure?

Do you have any written material about this procedure I can read?

Questions to ask once surgery is scheduled

Imagine that you are going to attend what could be the most important business meeting of your career. For the occasion, you are going to make a drastic change in your hair, such as having it permed or colored. The salon wants to schedule your appointment just prior to your business meeting. You have never met the stylist, and there will be no time for you to discuss what you want him to do. You realize that once you sit down in his chair, he will proceed immediately to perm or color your hair without any input from you. Would you agree to let this stranger work on your hair, or would you reschedule the appointment to give you enough time for a consultation first?

Now imagine that you are having surgery—not an emergency operation but a scheduled procedure. It is the day of surgery, and you have just been wheeled into the operating room. You are about to be put to sleep by a total stranger who has never spoken with you about the kind of anesthesia he will be using, or the risks involved, or asked you about any allergies or negative experiences you have previously had involving anesthesia. Would you let him go ahead and put you to sleep? If you would have rescheduled the hair appointment, why would you hesitate to insist that your surgery be rescheduled?

From my experience as a surgeon, I can say that the most important person in an operating room is the anesthesiologist. Once your gynecologist schedules you for surgery, he will call the anesthesiologist's office. "We're doing a laparoscopy on the twenty-third," he'll tell the secretary. A gynecologist almost never speaks directly to an anesthesiologist before surgery. That all-important member of your surgical team won't even know who you are unless you speak to him or her prior to the day of surgery.

Questions regarding anesthesia

It would be absurd for your anesthesiologist to meet you for the first time right before your surgery to ask whether you have any questions, when you might already be groggy from a preoperative sedative or anesthetic. That is why your anesthesiologist is obligated to phone or visit you the night before surgery to answer all your questions and to explain the anesthesiology consent form. If he does not contact you, exercise your right to refuse any preoperative sedation shot or pill until you meet with your anesthesiologist.

If the anesthesiologist won't take the time to explain everything thoroughly to you, insist that your surgery be rescheduled. Do not be concerned that your surgeon may have a friendly relationship with the anesthesiologist; your only concern should be acquiring enough information to make an informed choice to go ahead with anesthesia—just as you did when deciding on the surgery itself. There can be no surgery without you, so rest assured that if you decide to delay the surgery for a day or two, your doctor will still operate on you. Both you and your anesthesiologist should ask some vital questions.

Questions your anesthesiologist should ask you

What is your medical history?

Do you have any allergies?

Have you ever had any negative experiences with anesthesia?

Do you have any history of drug abuse?

Questions you should ask your anesthesiologist

What kind of anesthetic will you use: a local or regional (epidural, spinal), or general anesthetic?

What are the risks of the anesthesia?
    The risks of anesthesia will be listed on the anesthesia permit or consent form you will be asked to sign. It is the responsibility of the anesthesiologist to see that you give your written consent for anesthesia, although it is customary for a nurse to explain this form prior to surgery. However, the nurse won't be putting you to sleep, so insist that your anesthesiologist go over this form with you.

Please explain how the anesthesia will be administered.

Will I also be given a preoperative anesthetic or sedative?

Who will put me to sleep, you or a nurse?

Will any doctors-in-training be involved in administering the anesthetic?
It is your right to refuse to have doctors-in-training assisting your anesthesiologist.

Finally, assuming that you and your anesthesiologist have talked on the phone the night before surgery, he should also meet you in person the day of surgery, before you receive any preoperative sedation. You have had the chance to "sleep on" your conversation of the night before; this is your final opportunity to ask any questions that may still be on your mind.

Questions for your gynecologist

Will I be given an enema?

Can I eat or drink before surgery?

How will I feel after the operation?

What kind of pain will I feel right after surgery? Later on?

Is there anything I can do to help prevent some of this pain?
For example, constipation will aggravate the pain. To prevent this, ask your doctor if he will give you a stool softener to take before surgery.

What kind of pain medication can I take after the operation?
Ask your doctor to obtain this for you ahead of time, so you don't arrive home to find you don't have the pain medication you need.

Will I get to talk to you before the surgery?

I made a rule that no patient of mine would ever be taken to the operating room and put to sleep if I wasn't there to talk to her first. This is your absolute right: you must be allowed to meet with your gynecologist before he operates. Physicians aren't superhuman, and if your doctor was awake all night delivering three or four babies or handling some other emergency, he will be too tired to operate on you. So take a look at your doctor when he greets you before surgery. If he looks weary, ask whether he was up all night. Don't make the mistake of thinking he's a good doctor because he's so busy. You have the right to a surgeon who has had a full night's sleep. If your doctor looks too fatigued to operate, postpone the surgery.

Can my children visit me in the hospital before the operation? After the operation?

Within reason, I see no harm in your children visiting you, no matter how young they are. If you were close to them the day before surgery, sharing the same germs they have, what difference can it make if you see them again before and after the surgery? As long as you exercise good judgment, being with your family will probably do you—and them—a lot of good. Their presence won't make your doctor's job any harder, and if it helps alleviate your stress, it might even make it easier. Find out your hospital's policies on visitation before you are admitted and make the decision that is best for you, the consumer.

Will you be videotaping or taking pictures of my surgery?

Nearly all gynecological surgery is videotaped and photographed. Ask for copies of your video and pictures so you can discuss the outcome of your surgery with your gynecologist.

When I am in the hospital, will I be able to wear makeup (a wig, dentures, etc.)?

Patients can feel anxious before surgery because all of a sudden, they are not in control of their bodies. Everything revolves around what the doctor orders and what the nurses do. During this time little things such as being allowed to wear makeup can make a patient feel a lot better. Some hospitals make a fuss over this, but there is no medical reason to deny a patient this right.

What else can I do to prepare for surgery?

When it comes to surgery, often we women get in the way of our own recovery. We set ourselves up by doing almost everything around the house, so that even when we're going to have surgery, we don't ask for help at home. After surgery we are exhausted, but we go home and try to do too much, and so we don't heal as well as we could if we had the support and help of our families. For this reason, before one of my patients has surgery, I send home written instructions for the family. This tells them what mom should and should not do, and what I expect of them. Before major surgery, for example, someone should prepare and freeze at least two weeks of meals. No patient of mine is going to go home to cook for the family or schlep children around, for at least two weeks after surgery.

—Susan, a gynecologist and mother of three

Questions to ask after surgery

Sometimes after surgery, patients tell me, "I wanted to ask my doctor a few things, but he is always in and out of my room too fast. Either he'll knock on the door when I am in the shower, or he'll pop in and say he's on his way to surgery, and he disappears before I can say anything."

—Alice, a gynecological nurse

The care for which you are paying your doctor includes the postoperative time he spends with you explaining his findings, answering your questions, and outlining your post-operative care in a proper and timely fashion.

Is it proper and timely for your doctor to wait two days before he visits you? Is it acceptable for him to say a brief word to your family, then not see you until your follow-up appointment? Absolutely not. For one thing, when doctors tell family members things like "It's not cancer," anxious loved ones often remember only the word *cancer*. Most important, your family didn't have surgery, you did.

Right after you wake up (the newer anesthetics wear off fairly quickly), your doctor must pay you a short visit, even if you are a bit groggy. Will you comprehend everything your doctor has to tell you? Perhaps not, but at least you'll get the basics. Having had nine operations, I speak from experience. Even when I wasn't fully awake, I understood when a doctor told me that the operation had gone well.

Sometimes the diagnosis doesn't come back from the lab for several days. But your doctor can let you know whether everything went well, or that things don't look the way he hoped they would. His reassuring presence can be more important to you at that point than the diagnosis.

Questions for your doctor when you are fully awake from the anesthesia

What was the result of the operation?

How soon will you know whether the surgery was a success?

How soon can I go home?

After I am discharged, how soon do I need to see you again?

How long should it take before I feel completely recovered?

Can I take baths right away, or should I take showers instead?

How soon can I drive?

How soon can I go back to work?

Do I have to take any special care in lifting things?

Do I have to avoid certain kinds of exercise or sports? For how long?

Will I need to be on a special diet?

How soon can I use tampons?

How soon can I have sex?

My biggest gripe is that sex is seldom discussed before a patient is discharged. The doctor will tell her how soon she can bathe or drive, but a big part of this woman's life is not being addressed. She goes home thinking that she'll never be able to have sex again, but she's afraid to bring the subject up because she's afraid of what the doctor will think of her. Other patients have sex too early after surgery because the doctor didn't include this in his postoperative talk with her.

—Rene, a gynecological nurse

Overview of
surgical procedures

Biopsy

What is it?

A biopsy is the removal of a piece of tissue so it can be analyzed under a microscope. Gynecologists use biopsies in the evaluation of abnormal Pap smears (cervical biopsies), and lesions of the vagina and vulva (such as genital warts). Biopsies tell the doctor the degree of abnormality and, hopefully, its cause.

In what setting is it performed?

Biopsies are usually done in the doctor's office.

How long does the procedure take?

Five to ten minutes.

What kind of anesthetic is used?

A local anesthetic (numbing medicine such as Xylocaine applied to the biopsy site).

What is the usual recovery time?

Five to ten minutes.

When can I resume most normal activities (driving, working, exercising)?

Usually within the same day.

How soon can I resume sexual activity?

After a few days.

Cryotherapy

What is it?

Cryotherapy is treatment with an instrument that freezes and destroys abnormal tissue. A probe is used through which nitrous oxide is passed, freezing the tissue. It is frequently used to treat abnormal Pap smears.

In what setting is it performed?
A doctor's office.

How long does the procedure take?
Five to ten minutes.

What kind of anesthetic is used?
None is needed.

What is the usual recovery time?
Five to ten minutes.

When can I resume most normal activities (driving, working, exercising)?
The same day.

How soon can I resume sexual activity?
After two to three weeks.

Cauterization

What is it?

Cauterization is the delivery of an electric current to the tissue. Its applications include destruction of abnormal tissues in the vagina, cervix, and vulva. Its use in modern gynecology should be reserved for the destruction of external lesions such as vulvar genital warts.

In what setting is it performed?
A doctor's office.

How long does the procedure take?
Five to ten minutes.

What kind of anesthetic is used?
A local anesthetic.

What is the usual recovery time?
Five to ten minutes.

When can I resume most normal activities (driving, working, exercising)?
The same day.

How soon can I resume sexual activity?
After a few days.

Laser surgery

What is it?
A laser is a small, intense beam of electromagnetic energy used here as a surgical tool. It is used extensively in the treatment of cervical abnormalities such as dysplasia. It is also used for the removal of vaginal and vulvar lesions such as genital warts.

In what setting is it performed?
An office or operating room, depending on the extent of the abnormal area.

How long does the procedure take?
Fifteen to thirty minutes.

What kind of anesthetic is used?
A local or general anesthetic.

What is the usual recovery time?
Thirty minutes to a few hours.

When can I resume most normal activities (driving, working, exercising)?
The next day.

How soon can I resume sexual activity?
After a couple of weeks.

Cone biopsy of the cervix (conization)

What is it?
Conization is the surgical removal of a cone-shaped piece of tissue from the cervix and cervical canal and is used to diagnose or treat abnormalities of the cervix such as dysplasia. Physicians may use lasers, cauteries, or scalpels to perform this procedure. Cervical conization is rapidly being replaced by a new procedure called LLETZ (see below). Conization should be reserved for severe precancerous lesions or cancerous lesions.

In what setting is it performed?
Usually an operating room.

How long does the procedure take?
Thirty minutes.

What kind of anesthetic is used?
A general anesthestic.

What is the usual recovery time?
A few days.

When can I resume most normal activities (driving, working, exercising)?
After a few days.

How soon can I resume sexual activity?
After three to four weeks.

LLETZ (large loop excision of the transformation zone)

What is it?
LLETZ is a new gynecological procedure that has revolutionized the diagnosis and treatment of abnormal Pap smears. It has virtually eliminated the need for conization as we used to know it. It involves the use of a thin wire loop to remove a very shallow cone-shaped piece of the cervix. Its benefit over the cone biopsy is that it removes far less tissue, yet provides equal or better accuracy of diagnosis and/or treatment of the affected areas of the cervix. Scarring of the cervix is far less common than with the cone biopsy.

In what setting is it performed?
A doctor's office.

How long does the procedure take?
Five minutes.

What kind of anesthetic is used?
A local anesthetic.

What is the usual recovery time?
Fifteen to twenty minutes.

When can I resume most normal activities (driving, working, exercising)?
After thirty minutes.

How soon can I resume sexual activity?
After two to three weeks.

Laparoscopy

What is it?
Laparoscopy is a surgical procedure that allows the visualization of the pelvic organs: uterus, fallopian tubes, and ovaries. Through a small incision in the naval, the surgeon introduces a hollow fiberoptic instrument with a magnifying lens, called a laparoscope. Other even smaller incisions may be made in the lower abdomen. These allow instruments such as lasers, scissors, and biopsy forceps to be introduced into the abdomen. Laparoscopies may be used to identify or diagnose a particular problem, such as pelvic pain, or to treat various ailments.

Thanks to the advances of laparoscopy, gynecologists are able to perform extensive surgeries (such as hysterectomies and removal of the ovaries) through small incisions, instead of submitting the patient to old-style procedures requiring large incisions. At this time not all gynecologists are trained in the use of these complex laparoscopies, but there is always someone in proximity to you who is able to perform these procedures. Cysts "the size of a grapefruit" no longer require a six-inch incision in your abdomen; surprising as it may seem, they can usually be removed through a half-inch incision.

In what setting is it performed?
An operating room.

How long does the procedure take?
One to two hours.

What kind of anesthetic is used?
A general anesthetic.

What is the usual recovery time?
Two to four days.

When can I resume most normal activities (driving, working, exercising)?
After two to four days.

How soon can I resume sexual activity?
After seven to ten days.

Hysterectomy

What is it?
Hysterectomy is the surgical removal of the uterus, whether done vaginally, abdominally, or via a laparoscopy.

It is used to treat different ailments such as cancer of the uterus and/or cervix, severe menstrual bleeding, endometriosis, fibroids, and the complications of pelvic inflammatory disease.

In what setting is it performed?
An operating room.

How long does the procedure take?
One to two hours.

What kind of anesthetic is used?
A general or regional (spinal, epidural) anesthetic.

What is the usual recovery time?
Three to six weeks.

When can I resume most normal activities (driving, working, exercising)?
After three to six weeks.

How soon can I resume sexual activity?
After four to six weeks.

Oophorectomy

What is it?
Oophorectomy means the surgical removal of an ovary; bilateral oophorectomy indicates removal of both ovaries. The ovaries are olive-shaped glands connected by the fallopian tubes to the uterus. Ovaries secrete estrogen, which is the main female hormone. When one ovary is removed, the woman may produce enough estrogen with her remaining ovary to meet her body's needs. When both ovaries are removed, the woman will require hormone replacement (or

she will begin to experience symptoms of menopause). Oophorectomies are used for treatment of ovarian tumors, cysts, endometriosis, pelvic inflammatory disease, and ovarian cancers. They may be done through a traditional abdominal incision or through more modern laparoscopic techniques.

In what setting is it performed?
An operating room.

How long does the procedure take?
One to two hours.

What kind of anesthetic is used?
A general anesthetic.

What is the usual recovery time?
Two to three weeks.

When can I resume most normal activities (driving, working, exercising)?
After two weeks.

How soon can I resume sexual activity?
After two to three weeks.

PART FIVE

CHAPTER 17

Prevention:
What Are Your Options?

Are you perplexed about safe, safer, safest sex?

In the wake of the epidemic of sexually transmitted diseases (STDs), everyone has something to say about prevention. Some voices moralize, some lecture, some keep to the safe middle ground, some rationalize, some shout a warning, some attempt to rally a call to action. What can I possibly add? Straight talk from a gynecologist, the solid information you need to make the choices that are right for you.

First I'm going to take off my white coat briefly and let you in on some of the feelings I might usually keep to myself or only share with a colleague. It has always been part of a physician's lot to deal with the sadness and helplessness of seeing patients suffer from diseases we don't fully understand and cannot cure; but can you imagine the frustration and anger a gynecologist feels when he or she sees a patient die from a disease that was caused by sex— a disease that could have been prevented?

There is no such thing as absolutely safe sex, other than abstaining until marriage, marrying another virgin or someone who has been tested and shown to be noninfected, then staying married and mutually faithful for life. Even your safety within marriage rests on the integrity of the other person. Neither of you can ever forget that it only takes one sexual act with an infected third party to introduce an STD into your marriage, and that no method of protection is 100 percent effective.

Keeping all the risks in mind, if you still choose to be sexually active, then you need to know your options. Casual, unprotected sex is out of the question. You know that by now or you would not be reading this chapter. So let us assume that—with your eyes wide open—you are choosing to be sexually active at this time. Have you also made a firm decision to protect yourself to the best of your ability? I know it is unfair that the responsibility for sexual protection should fall entirely on your shoulders, but with the exception of AIDS, women who choose to be sexually active run a greater risk than men—from unwanted pregnancy to infertility to death. A man can have an STD, pass it on to all his partners, and never experience one symptom. For that reason, fair or not, it is your responsibility to yourself to safeguard your own health.

Where do you start? Picture a four-legged table. Just as this table would be useless if it were missing a leg, any plan you have to practice the safest sex possible will fail if it does not include each of the following elements. You must:

1. Have regular gynecological checkups including Pap smears, and insist that you be screened for STDs.
2. Avoid risky sexual practices.
3. Use protection methods the proper way every time you have sex.
4. Choose your partners wisely.

Let's examine these points more closely:

1. Have regular gynecological checkups including Pap smears, and insist that you be screened for STDs.

Remember that sexually transmitted disease is primarily a silent disease; there are few symptoms to tip you off to an infection either in your partner or in yourself. Regular gynecological exams can screen you for the consequences of some STDs, but as yet most gynecologists do not routinely test all patients for the most widespread STDs. However, your doctor will ask questions about your sexual practices to help gauge the possibility that you have been exposed to an STD. Help him to help you by answering thoroughly and honestly and by insisting that he test you regularly for common STDs. Learn as much as you can on your own about STDs, so that you can make the best use of your gynecologist as a resource to answer your remaining questions.

2. Avoid risky sexual practices.

- Avoid any unprotected sexual activities, including intercourse and oral sex. Any unprotected sexual activity in which you and your partner exchange bodily fluids—especially semen, vaginal and cervical secretions, and blood—must be considered high risk.
- Avoid anal sex. Anal sex is the riskiest method of intercourse because blood vessels lining the anus and rectum are easy to rupture, giving infectious agents a direct passageway to the bloodstream.
- Avoid oral-anal contact.
- Avoid the use of alcohol and other drugs, which may lower your inhibitions and affect your judgment, leaving you more likely to engage in unsafe sexual practices.

Consider sensual activities that don't require a condom:
- Massage
- Petting
- Hugging and rubbing bodies together
- Masturbating your partner
- Self-masturbation

3. Use protection the proper way every time you have sex.

The condom is the best method available for the prevention of sexually transmitted diseases. To increase protection, use a condom with another barrier method, such as a diaphragm or sponge in combination with a spermicide. Birth control pills do not provide any protection against sexually transmitted diseases.

How to select and store a condom:
- DO use high-quality latex, reservoir (nipple)-tip, lubricated-type condoms only. These are available in different textures, colors, and sometimes in different sizes.
- DO buy prelubricated condoms containing nonoxynol-9, a chemical barrier that may reduce your chances of contracting some STDs.
- DO store condoms in a cool, dry place.

- DON'T buy condoms made of any material other than latex. So-called natural membranes or animal skins contain pores that the HIV virus can easily pass through.
- DON'T buy or use condoms past the expiration date on the outer package.
- DON'T store condoms in your car's glove compartment; they can be damaged by heat.
- DON'T carry condoms in a wallet for long periods of time; this shortens their shelf life.
- DON'T ever reuse a condom.

How to use a condom:

- DO use condoms for the first six months of any sexual relationship. If your partner has been exposed to the HIV virus, it can take up to six months before his body produces enough antibodies to test positive for HIV.
- DO roll the condom down on the penis as soon as it is erect, before you begin foreplay or intercourse.
- DO leave 1/4-1/2 inch of extra space at the tip of the condom to catch the semen if the condom does not have a reservoir end.
- DO use a water-based lubricant, such as spermicidal jelly, if you are using nonlubricated condoms.
- DO hold the condom at the rim and remove soon after ejaculation while your partner's penis is still hard.
- DO wrap the used condom in tissue and dispose of it safely.

- DON'T wait until just before penetration to put a condom on. Even before ejaculation, the penis can leak fluid and semen that can infect you with an STD or impregnate you.
- DON'T unroll the condom before putting it on the penis; instead, carefully roll it on all the way toward the base of the penis.
- DON'T use oil-based lubricants such as petroleum jelly (Vaseline) or vegetable oil; these can damage condoms.
- DON'T wait to remove the condom until your partner's penis goes soft inside you; it may come off, and protection would be lost.
- DON'T tug the condom off, as it may tear.
- DON'T allow semen to come into contact with any wound or broken skin, or to spill on your hands or body. Wash your hands or other body parts if contact occurs.

The female condom is receiving much publicity but, as of yet, has not made a big impact on the prevention of STDs. A latex pouch with a ring at its closed end is inserted into the vagina and pushed upward toward the cervix. A ring at the open end remains outside the body. This pouch prevents semen from coming into contact with the labia, vagina, or cervix, therefore protecting against pregnancy and STDs. There are conflicting reports on the rate of failure (due to breakage or slippage) of this condom. Time will tell whether or not society will embrace the use of a female condom.

4. Choose your sexual partners wisely.
- DON'T go to bed with a man who uses IV drugs.
- DON'T go to bed with a man who won't use a condom.
- DON'T go to bed with a man unless you are sure he has tested negative for STDs.
- DON'T go to bed with a man unless you and he have a monogamous relationship.
- DON'T go to bed with a man if he shows any symptoms of an STD, such as difficulty urinating, a discharge from his penis, or a bump or sore on his genitals.

Questions to ask your partner about high-risk activities

Have you been tested for HIV and other STDs?

How many sex partners have you had over the last five years?

Have you ever had sex with a prostitute?

Have you ever had sex with another man? (About 15 percent of the male population has had a same-sex experience.)

Have you or your previous partners ever injected drugs? If so, did you share needles?

Have you ever had a blood transfusion (especially before 1985, when blood wasn't screened for HIV)?

CHAPTER 18

If I Could Talk to Your Doctor

Straight talk from one gynecologist to another

Every day a newspaper or magazine prints another feature story on the health care profession. Most focus on the rift in trust between patients and doctors; patients feel that we as physicians no longer listen to them. Gynecologists are a main target of this criticism. As we read these articles, deep in our hearts we know they are right. For whatever reason and in spite of our excuses, we have lost the human touch. We don't talk to our patients, we don't listen. Sometimes we are in a hurry, sometimes we forget, sometimes we think we talked to them; but the bottom line is, our patients don't think we are doing a good job—and I agree with them.

I have written this book so that patients may better understand issues that concern them. The book is not intended to diminish the doctor's role; on the contrary, it will strengthen the doctor-patient relationship by creating avenues of communication. As a teacher, I see bright and highly skilled gynecologists-in-training who still refer to patients as "that hysterectomy" or "that abnormal Pap smear." It's as if they are afraid to get close to their patients, to get to know them, to hold their hand, to listen. It's your responsibility to understand that listening is just as important a skill as having a steady scalpel.

Every gynecologist has seen a patient in his or her practice who didn't understand why certain procedures were done to her. Instead of calling those patients difficult when they ask us questions, it is time we sit down with them and educate them as we should have done in the first place.

If your patient has an STD, tell her—don't beat around the bush by calling it "a little infection." If she has an abnormal Pap smear, explain its cause in language she will understand. Having your nurse call the patient with the results is not what the patient paid you for. As medical director of women's clinics for the last nine years, I have called an average of 150 patients per month with abnormal Pap smear results. The average gynecologist may encounter ten abnormal Pap smears a month. So the excuse "I'm too busy" doesn't fly. Women who have read this book now know that doctors—not nurses—should explain test results and answer questions. If you, as a doctor, choose to continue with the status quo, before long you *will* have time to call because you won't be busy.

When a patient desires a second opinion, encourage her; don't put obstacles in her way. Make her records accessible to her. Don't make her feel she's being "unfaithful" to you. Remember that a well-informed patient is the best patient to have. If her second-opinion doctor suggests a newer procedure that you don't feel technically comfortable with—encourage her if it's in her best interests—to go ahead with that alternative. Instead of complaining, go and learn that newer technique. And if you are giving a second opinion, be honest enough to disagree with your colleague, even if you're going to play golf with him on Saturday.

I find it interesting that when my wife goes to her gynecologist, they treat her with kid gloves and spend hours explaining her condition; but when a woman who has no connection with gynecology, either directly or indirectly, goes to her doctor, she is given only a few rushed minutes. The technical words we use are mind-boggling to her. Unlike my wife, who can ask me questions twenty-four hours a day, this woman has only those few minutes to get all her questions answered. An inquisitive patient is not trying to take over your practice or tell you what to do; she's trying to find out what's going on—that's her responsibility as a patient.

In the operating room, we make sure the incision looks pretty because that's all the patient will see. Now we find ourselves with a patient who demands to understand what happened below the skin. There's no excuse not to accommodate her. Nearly every hospital has the capacity to produce videos and still photos instantaneously. Show them to your patient and give her copies to take home. Explain what was done in language that is clear.

I know I have opened a can of worms with this book. Maybe, for whatever reason, you didn't explain to your patient what her abnormal Pap smear really meant. Now is the time to do so. Let's establish a new relationship and a new trust between ourselves and our patients. If you think that Mary will commit suicide if you tell her in plain English that she has an STD, then you don't belong in gynecology.

When I go to the car shop, I am amused by the sign that reads "No customers allowed in the work area." I barge in without hesitation and beleaguer the poor mechanic with questions. Low and behold, the last time that happened, I realized he was putting the wrong motor oil in my car. Gynecologists' office have replaced the "keep out" sign with frosted glass at the receptionist's window to create an air of mystique and an atmosphere of "us" and "them." We treat our patients as if we are adults and they are children, instead of welcoming them as our partners in health care and our clients in business.

Realize that all the educational material in the world, such as videos and written literature, pale in comparison to your words and understanding. I have never permitted a patient education room in my offices. *I* do the educating. Our goal is the same as the patient's: to achieve a cure and/or minimize the damage done by disease. However, doctors cannot do this alone. We need the patient's support and understanding, which can only be accomplished through education.

The partnership between patient and doctor that I outline in this book will benefit everyone. It will result in better medicine, and it will result in fewer visits for a recurrent problem. Patients are consumers, and they will choose the doctor who listens and shows he or she cares.

APPENDIX

A Word to Young Women

Your first gynecological exam

If you are a young woman who hasn't spent much, if any, time in a gynecologist's office, you probably have needs and questions that deserve special attention. I'd like to share some straight talk with you as though I am a doctor you are meeting for the first time and this is your first visit to a gynecologist. Some of the things I have to say won't fit your situation, but they all come from the many talks I have had with my younger patients. I hope that reading this will help you feel comfortable enough to ask the questions that are on your mind when you go to see your own gynecologist.

Right off, I want you to know that everything you tell a doctor is private. Even if your mom or dad brought you here, everything we talk about is just between you and me, if that is what you want. Also, you get to choose whether or not we talk in private. Let's imagine that your mom came with you. We can ask her to leave the room or she can stay—whatever is comfortable for you. But please understand that I'm going to ask some serious questions, and some of them might embarrass you. For example, I'll have to know whether you have had sex, and I'll need you to be absolutely honest. If you might not be able to answer my questions in front of your mom, let me know. I'll help her to understand that we need to talk in private.

You have a right to talk to me in my office with your clothes on *before* I begin your physical exam. At some gynecologists' offices, a nurse may weigh you, check your pulse, or do other simple tests before you undress to see the doctor. That's okay, but if a gynecologist ever wants you to get undressed before you have a talk, tell him you won't be able to concentrate unless you can talk in his office with your clothes *on*. You might want to have your mom check on this when she calls to make your appointment.

Just about every young woman who comes for her first gynecological exam is scared and embarrassed, so you probably won't be any different. It will help you feel better if you can trust me enough to tell me your fears. What horrible things have you heard about going to the gynecologist? If you are really nervous about having a pelvic exam, let me know. I'll do whatever I can to help you relax. The talking we'll do is the most important part of your first visit to a gynecologist, so perhaps we can just get to know one another for now, and you can come back another time for your physical exam.

Let's assume, though, that you are going to have the entire exam today. You have the right to ask me to explain everything I am going to do and why it will help you. I'm not going to consider any of your questions stupid. Feel free to ask about anything—birth control, having periods, what to do about cramps and acne, how to use tampons, whether your breast size is normal, and about any diseases you could get by having sex. I don't want to scare you, but you need to know that you could get into a lot of trouble if you don't have the right information.

If you're already sexually active, what about your boyfriend? He needs to hear what I have to say, too. Does he know that a guy might catch a disease from having sex and not even know he had it? I'm not just talking about AIDS. I'm also going to tell you about other sexually transmitted diseases (we call them STDs). A lot of STDs usually don't harm a guy, but without meaning to, he could infect his girlfriend during sex, and that STD could do a lot of damage inside her before she knew that anything was wrong. How do we know that your boyfriend didn't catch something from his previous girlfriend and pass it on to you? If you're going to take on the responsibility of having sex, your boyfriend needs to share that responsibility fifty-fifty. I'll be happy to suggest where he can get some of the same tests I'm going to give you, to make sure both of you are healthy.

After we trade questions and answers for a while, I'm going to walk you through the steps of the exam. I'll explain all the tests that the nurse will do and why we make you wear such a skimpy gown. In the examining room, I'll show you the examining table and explain why you need to scoot down and put your feet in the stirrups during the exam. If you want, I'll show you the instruments I'll be using.

The nurse will be in the room with us during the exam. She's there to help you understand what is going on; don't be embarrassed to ask her to hold your hand—she does that all the time. I won't mind if you feel like asking her any questions you think are too embarrassing to share with me. Also, it doesn't make you a wimp if you would like your mom in the room—or a horrible person if you ask her to leave. This is your exam, and it's your choice.

Once you've seated yourself on the examining table, I will start by examining you in some of the ways that other doctors do, such as pressing gently on your throat, neck, and stomach. If my hands are cold, let me know so I can warm them. When I examine your breasts, instead of being embarrassed, pay attention to what I do. I will show you how to do this yourself every month.

Then you'll scoot all the way down to the end of the table and put your feet in the stirrups. I'll put some gloves on and touch the outside of your body. If you want, I'll hold up a mirror and explain anything you don't understand about the parts of your body. Please don't be embarrassed to ask me to show you things like the lips of your vagina or your clitoris. This is a doctor's office, and to me it's no different than looking at your toes. I want you to know about your body so you can be proud of it and know how to take care of it.

Then I'll put a small speculum inside your vagina. If you are a virgin, there are ways I can do the exam that won't take away your virginity. I can use a very small speculum that you will hardly feel. Remember too that a lot of active young women don't have a hymen (a little membrane that partially covers the vagina), but they are still virgins. You could have ridden a horse or a bicycle so vigorously that you no longer have a hymen, even though you are still a virgin.

When I put in the speculum, you may feel uncomfortable. If it hurts, tell me and I'll use a smaller one. I will also warm it up. You may notice a little spotting after you get home, but this is normal.

Now I'll do all those tests that we already talked about in my office, such as the Pap smear, or tests for STDs. You can keep asking me questions, and everything you say will be just between us.

After the examination is over, we'll talk some more. If you want me to put you on birth control pills, I'll explain their pros and cons and the responsibility that goes with taking them. We'll talk about what I found during your exam. Now that you can relax, you can ask some of the questions that you may have been holding back.

Let me give you one example. I had a patient who was embarrassed to tell me that she put a tampon in and couldn't get it out. Well, those things happen. Sometimes women even forget to take one tampon out before putting another in. But this young woman left it in too long, and she almost died from a disease called toxic shock syndrome. It's a disease you can get if you don't know how to use a tampon properly. Gynecologists can help you with things like that.

You may already have a gynecologist you're seeing. If you feel he doesn't listen, or if you feel that he is judging you, leave. There are plenty of us who are not going to judge you. There are plenty of us who will teach you how to prevent problems rather than just treating them.

Remember, you have to help your doctor to help you. Open up to your doctor. If you're going to allow him to examine you in a very private part of your body, let him ask you personal questions. Don't tell him that you're not having sex if you are. Tell him if you have more than one partner. He needs all that information so he can help you have a happy and healthy sex life, and help ensure that you're able to have children later on if you want them. Be honest with your answers—it could save your life.

Glossary

ABDOMEN – a cavity in the body containing organs such as the stomach, intestines, and liver

ABSCESS – pus accumulated from broken-down tissue

ABSTINENCE – doing without voluntarily; *see* Celibacy

ACQUIRED IMMUNE DEFICIENCY SYNDROME – *see* AIDS

ACUTE – highly sensitive; or sudden, sharp (as of pain)

ACYCLOVIR – antiviral drug used in the treatment of herpes infections

AIDS (ACQUIRED IMMUNE DEFICIENCY SYNDROME) – a condition, eventually fatal, in which the immune system fails to provide normal protection from infection

ALLERGY – hypersensitivity to a substance

ANALGESIC – a substance that relieves pain; e.g., aspirin

ANEMIA – a deficiency in the hemoglobin content of the blood often caused by insufficient iron in the diet; symptoms are fatigue, weakness, and headaches

ANESTHESIA – a general or local loss of feeling induced by disease or drugs

ANESTHETIC – a pain-relieving drug

ANTIBIOTIC – a drug (such as penicillin) that slows the growth of, or destroys, certain bacteria; used to treat infectious diseases

ANTIBODY – a protein in the blood that neutralizes an antigen to help the body destroy invading microorganisms

ANTIFUNGAL – an agent destructive of fungi; e.g., Monistat

ANTIGEN – a substance that stimulates the production of antibodies in the body's defense against infection and disease

ANTIVIRAL – a drug destructive of viruses

ANUS – the opening in the rectum through which feces are excreted

ARTHRITIS – inflammation of a joint or joints

ASYMPTOMATIC – free from symptoms

AZT (AZIDOTHYMIDINE) – *see* Zidovudine

BACTERIAL CULTURE – *see* culture

BACTERIUM – one of the various microscopic organisms that cause disease

BARTHOLIN'S GLAND – one of two small glands on either side of the vaginal opening that secrete mucus; easily infected and may become painfully swollen and abscessed

BENIGN – harmless; not malignant

BIOPSY – microscopic examination of tissues or fluids removed from the body

BIRTH CONTROL – *see* Contraception

BISEXUAL – sexually attracted to both men and women

BLADDER – the urinary bladder serves as the storage for urine

BLISTER – a swelling on the skin or mucous surface filled with fluid

BLOOD TEST – a test to analyze the structure and makeup of the blood; e.g., test for syphilis

BOIL – a pus-filled inflammation of the skin

BOWEL – all or part of the intestines

BREAST EXAMINATION – the examination of the breast to detect changes (such as lumps) that may indicate the onset of disease

CANCER – a malignant growth of cells

CANDIDA ALBICANS – the fungus that causes candidiasis

CANDIDIASIS – a common fungal infection of the vagina (also the skin or mouth)

CARRIER – one who harbors an infectious disease that can be transmitted to others, but who may enjoy some immunity and freedom from symptoms

CAUTERIZATION – tissue destruction by burning or searing with an electric spark, a heated instrument, or by application of a caustic agent

CELIBACY – the state of being unmarried; more commonly, abstinence from sexual intercourse

CERVICAL CANCER – a malignant tumor of the cervix

CERVICITIS – fungal, bacterial, viral, or other infection of the cervix

CERVIX – the neck of the uterus

CESAREAN SECTION – the surgical delivery of a baby through the abdomen

CHANCRE – a sore usually with a hard rim or base; esp. the primary sore of syphilis

CHANCROID – a painful genital ulcer

CHLAMYDIA TRICHOMATIS – a microscopic organism that commonly causes urethritis, cervicitis, and pelvic inflammatory disease

CHRONIC – of long duration or of frequent recurrence

CLITORIS – a small, highly sensitive erectile structure situated near the urethral opening in the female

COITUS – sexual intercourse

COLON – part of the large intestine leading from the small intestine to the rectum

COLPOSCOPE – a magnifying instrument enabling the visual examination of the vagina and/or cervix

CONDOM – a tubular sheath fitted over the penis to reduce the chance of infection and/or conception during sexual intercourse

CONTAGIOUS – capable of disease transmission by direct or indirect contact

CONTRACEPTION – the intentional avoidance of conception; birth control

CONTRACT – to acquire an infection or disease

CRYOSURGERY – surgery performed by the freezing of tissue

CULTURE – the growing of microorganisms for scientific study or medicinal use; a laboratory test to identify and grow organisms related to an infection

CYSTITIS – inflammation of the bladder caused by an infection

DIAPHRAGM – a contraceptive dome made of rubber that fits over the cervix to prevent pregnancy

DISEASE – an abnormal condition caused by infection, poor diet, tumors, or other injurious mechanisms

DOXYCYCLINE – an antibiotic used in the treatment of pelvic inflammatory disease

ECTOPIC PREGNANCY – a pregnancy developing outside the uterus

ENDOMETRITIS – inflammation of the lining of the uterus usually caused by a bacterial infection

ENDOMETRIUM – the mucous membrane lining of the uterus

EPIDIDYMIS – a cordlike mass on the back surface of the testicle

EPIDIDYMITIS – inflammation of the epididymis

ERYTHROMYCIN – an antibiotic drug used in the treatment of genital infections

ESTROGEN – the female sex hormone produced in the ovaries

EXCISION – the surgical removal of a body part

FALLOPIAN TUBE – one of two tubes transporting the egg, or ovum, from the ovary to the uterus

FERTILE – capable of conceiving

FIMBRIA – the open end of the fallopian tube

FLAYGL – the trade name of a drug (metronidazole) used to treat vaginal infections

FUNGUS – an organism which causes disease, such as a vaginal infection

GARDNERELLA VAGINALIS – a bacteria that causes nonspecific vaginitis

GENITAL HERPES – a painful viral infection occurring in the genital area

GENITAL TRACT – the region of the body containing parts related to the reproductive process

GENITAL WART – a viral lesion on the male or female genitals

GENITALIA – the external reproductive organs of males or females

GLANS CLITORIS – the head of the clitoris

GLANS PENIS – the head of the penis

GONAD – the organ that generates reproductive cells (ovary or testicle)

GONOCOCCUS – the bacteria that causes gonorrhea

GONORRHEA – a sexually transmitted disease that can lead to widespread infections and disorders, including pelvic inflammatory disease

GRANULOMA INGUINALE – a chronic and progressive sexually transmitted disease characterized by ulcers in the genital and groin regions

GROIN – the space between the thigh and the lower abdomen

HAEMOPHILUS DUCREYI – the bacteria that causes chancroid

HBV (HEPATITIS B VIRUS) – a virus that causes a liver inflammation

HEMOGLOBIN – a molecular compound in red blood cells that carries oxygen to body tissues

HEMORRHAGE – the profuse and rapid loss of blood

HEPATITIS – inflammation of the liver

HETEROSEXUAL – a person who engages in sexual activity with a member of the opposite sex

HIV (HUMAN IMMUNODEFICIENCY VIRUS) – the AIDS virus

HOMOSEXUAL – a person who engages in sexual activity with a member of the same sex

HORMONE – a complex substance carried by body fluids that regulates the activity of specific organs or tissues; e.g., estrogen, progesterone, and testosterone

HPV (HUMAN PAPILLOMA VIRUS) – the microorganism that causes genital warts and lesions of the cervix

HYSTERECTOMY – the surgical removal of the uterus

IMMUNE – highly resistant to, or protected from, a disease

IMMUNODEFICIENCY – a lacking in the body's antibody system, lowering resistance to infection and/or disease

INCIDENCE – the number of occurrences in a specific period of time

INCUBATION PERIOD – the time between infection and the first symptom of disease

INFECT – to transmit a disease

INFECTION – a disease caused by the invasion of a pathogen (a microscopic organism) into the body

INFECTIOUS – capable of communicating disease

INFERTILE – incapable of conceiving

INFLAMMATION – localized swelling, redness, heat, and pain of body tissues responding to irritation, infection, or injury

INTERCOURSE – a sexual coupling

IUD (INTRAUTERINE DEVICE) – a small device that is inserted into the uterus for continuous contraception

IV (INTRAVENOUS) – into a vein

JAUNDICE – the yellowing of the skin and of the whites of the eyes (usually caused by hepatitis)

KWELL – the trade name of an insecticide (lindane) used to treat infestations of lice and mites

LABIUM – each of the large outer, and small inner, edges of the female external genitalia

LIVER – the large glandular organ located in the abdomen that performs many complex body functions

LYMPH – a yellowish tissue fluid that circulates through lymph nodes into the blood stream

LYMPH NODE – a small cluster of cells that are part of the body's cellular defenses

LYMPHOGRANULOMA VENEREUM – a sexually transmitted disease caused by the bacteria *Chlamydia trachomatis*

MALIGNANT – a cancer that spreads, causing death

MENSTRUAL FLOW – the flow of blood during menstruation

MICROORGANISM – a unicellular living organism; e.g., a bacteria, virus, fungus

MOLLUSCUM – a disease of the skin usually appearing in round, soft masses

MONILIASIS – a vaginal yeast infection

MONS PUBIS – the rounded prominence in the lower female abdomen just above the external female genitalia

MUCOPURULENT – a mixture of mucous and pus

NEISSERIA GONORRHOEAE – *see* Gonococcus

NONOXYNOL-9 – a chemical used as a spermicide

NONSPECIFIC INFECTION – an infection, often of the genitalia, caused by a microorganism that is neither gonorrhoeae nor chlamydia

OOPHORECTOMY – the excision of one or both ovaries

ORAL – relating to the mouth

ORGAN – a body part having a specific function, such as the heart or lungs

ORGANISM – any form of life, such as an animal or a plant; microscopically, a cell, bacteria, or virus

OVARY – one of two female reproductive organs that produce eggs

OVIDUCT – the tube through which the ovum, or egg, passes; (see Fallopian Tube)

OVULATION – the escape of an egg from the ovary

PAP SMEAR – *see* Papanicolaou test

PAPANICOLAOU TEST – a test for the early detection of cervical cancer

PEDICULOSIS PUBIS – the formal name of an infestation of crab lice

PELVIC INFLAMMATORY DISEASE (PID) – an inflamed condition of the female reproductive organs

PELVIS – the cavity in the lower part of the trunk of the body

PENICILLIN – an antibiotic used to treat bacterial infections

PENIS – the male organ of copulation and urination

PERINEUM – the space between the anus and the vulva in females

PID – *see* Pelvic inflammatory disease

PODOPHYLLIN – a resin used as a topical caustic in the treatment of genital warts

PROGESTERONE – a female sex hormone

PROMISCUITY – frequent and careless sexual activity; statistically enhances the chance of contracting a disease

PROPHYLACTIC – a disease-preventive measure or medicine; e.g., a condom

PROSTATE GLAND – a glandular organ in the male located at the base of the bladder that produces the fluid part of semen

PROSTATITIS – inflammation of the prostate gland

PUS – a yellowish white fluid occurring at an infection site

PUSTULE – a blister-like elevation of the skin containing pus

RASH – an eruption of red spots on the skin

RECTUM – the terminal portion of the large intestine connecting the colon and the anus

RETROVIR – the trade name for AZT

RETROVIRUS – a member of a large group of infectious agents that cause AIDS

Salpingitis – an infection of the fallopian tube

Semen – the fluid discharge in ejaculation

Sexual intercourse – the insertion of the penis into the vagina

Sexually transmitted disease (STD) – a disease that is transmitted by sexual contact

Speculum – a dilating instrument used for the examination of the vagina

Sperm – the male reproductive cell conveyed in semen

Spermicide – a substance or agent that kills sperm

STD – *see* Sexually transmitted disease

Sterile – incapable of producing offspring

Subclinical – a manifestation of a disease too mild for detection by normal tests

Surgery – the instrumental, incisional, or manual treatment of bodily disorders and injuries

Symptoms – the subjective indication of a disease

Syphilis – an infectious disease caused by invasion of a spirochete

Testis – either of two male sex or reproductive glands that produce sperm; located in the scrotum

Testosterone – the principal male sex hormone produced in the testis

Treponema pallidum – the spirochete that causes syphilis

Trichomoniasis – a vaginal infection

Tubal pregnancy – a fertilized egg developing in one of the fallopian tubes

Ulcer – an open sore

Urethra – the tube by which urine is discharged from the bladder

Urethritis – inflammation of the urethra

Uterus – the womb

Vagina – the passage in the female situated between the uterus and the vulva

Vaginitis – inflammation of the vagina

Vulva – the external part of the female genitalia

Zidovudine – an antiviral drug used in the treatment of AIDS

Information Resources

National STD Hotline
1-800-227-8922 (toll-free)
Gives information on all sexually transmitted diseases.

National AIDS Hotline
1-800-342-2437 (toll-free)
Provides information about AIDS and gives referrals to local groups for further services.

TTY/TTD Hotline (for hearing-impaired persons)
1-800-AIDS-TTY (toll-free)

American College Health Association
P.O. Box 28937
Baltimore, MD 21240-8937
(410) 859-1500
Informative pamphlets on safer sex and AIDS.

American College of Obstetricians and Gynecologists Resource Center
Suite 300 East
600 Maryland Ave SW
Washington, DC 20024

National Women's Health Network
224 7th Street SE
Washington, DC 20003

Other sources of help and information:
Your local or state public health department
Your doctor
Your library